# THE ROYAL COLLEGE OF SAN CARLOS

*To Kathy, Tracey, David, and Stephen*

# THE ROYAL COLLEGE OF SAN CARLOS

*Surgery and Spanish Medical Reform in the Late Eighteenth Century*

MICHAEL E. BURKE

DUKE UNIVERSITY PRESS
DURHAM, N. C.
1977

L.C.C. card number 76–50237
ISBN 0–8223–0382–5

Printed in the United States of America
by Heritage Printers, Inc.

## Contents

# Foreword

Here is a book by a young man with a natural grasp of a truth that escapes too many far older foreign observers commenting on Spain: that both tradition and the urge to change, even when they were in direct conflict, somehow acted upon each other to advance science in Spain. In the first half of the eighteenth century, the chief critic of backward medicine in the country, Fray Benito Jerónomo de Feijóo (1676–1764), in his own person combined these seeming contradictions in high degree. So did Antonio Gimbernat, the founder of San Carlos. Though he had many of the typical failings of the scholastic academic at that late date, he nevertheless enlisted the support of the government for the College. This success, in fact, was all but epoch-making, for the slowness of Spain in expanding and modernizing higher education in science was owing to nothing so much as to want of money. And the sanction of the government meant more certain financing. Gimbernat's ally, the Count of Campomanes (1723–1802), a central and uncompromising exponent of the Enlightenment, was ideally placed as fiscal (crown attorney) of the Council of Castile. The Count's tack was not only to admit but to emphasize the widespread ignorance and charlantry in ordinary Spanish medicine and surgery. The new academies and societies, searching for the "useful," took the practical, the pragmatic approach. Thus, the advance from tradition in Spain was more than a sudden burst of light late in the eighteenth century.

But beneath the agitation for reform that issued from the mouths of famous men such as Feijóo and Campomanes there was a quiet realization among all ordinary educated men that they must face scientific problems with Descartes's "methodical doubt," and proceed through "observation" and the "evidence of the senses," yet with Descartes's vortexes they would have nothing to do. This proof that they distrusted "systems" in science—the bête noire of medical progress—shows how close to intellectual maturity they were. That in medical science they did not, by the same tenent, reject blood-letting shows how tenuous and delicate was this victory—not just in Spain but everywhere. In Spanish universities, medicine remained on the bottom rung of precedence. Law students still outnumbered those in medicine five to one.

The low repute of the medical professions among aristocrats is, then, reflected by the scarcity of doctors. Qualification to practice required a candidate to have a medical degree—baccalaureate, licentiate, or doctorate—from a designated Spanish university and a certificate showing that he had successfully passed examination by the Royal Protomedicato. A young man, though he might attend the university and qualify to practice as a "Latin surgeon," knew that for this kind of academic effort he could acquire far greater prestige with the title of physician. The result was that Romancistas (surgeons trained by the apprenticeship method), phlebotomists, and plain *curanderos* took over practice—when anybody did. Across the seas in America the shortage of certified doctors and surgeons remained chronic, with all the ills flowing from such a glaring and universal want. Mexico City, the metropolis of the New World, a quarter of a century after the Conquest, had only two licensed doctors, with one of them himself sick. At the time of Francisco Xavier Balmis's celebrated vaccinating expedition to America in 1804 many cities and some provincial capitals still had no doctors at all. Of the countryside there is no need to speak.

To meet a situation like this one of two courses might be taken. The first was to give more young men—inevitably of the lower classes—some training in the treatment of the most common diseases and in the most elementary surgical procedures. This course, because it seemed to be a compromise with the unrealistic standards of the Protomedicato (Board of King's Physicians) and in violation of the statutes of the universities, never got beyond the stage of being proposed, in America at least, by three or four people. The creation of modern surgical colleges to train a number of surgeons by the highest standards to serve as models for others was the second answer, the one that the Spaniards tried to follow. The colleges founded—in Cádiz (1748), Barcelona (1764), and Madrid (1787)—symbolize this new outlook. The modern philosophy and agitation necessary to launch and sustain all three of them inevitably inclined the Spanish government to sanction independent surgical education in America also. The Academy of Surgery in the Royal Indian Hospital in Mexico City, approved in 1768, was the one tangible result in the eighteenth century. In this process, the physicians in both Spain and America began to fall behind, vexed and bewildered to have mere surgeons scorn their backwardness.

The founders of San Carlos in Madrid, their national pride touched, had the insight and the willingness—even eagerness—to profit by foreign progress in surgery. In fact, they flung open the doors so wide as to invite foreign empirics (*intrusos*) to enter too. Besides those who went abroad on their own, official delegations traveled outside the country to keep up with the latest in "studies," surgical techniques, and even instruments. As this was an age of the expert craftsman, the College of San Carlos brought in its own instrument-maker and willy nilly became a kind of national pool for surgical instruments. When an officious individual offered to bring together in San Carlos a collection of wax anatomical figures equal to that "in Berlin," the faculty responded with disdain that, to match any collection, all it needed was money. Besides, anatomy minute and realistic enough to benefit the truly modern surgeon had to be gained by dissecting the human body, and not by reading Winslow's *Anatomical Exposition*—the text assigned—and the Gray's *Anatomy* of that day.

To treat this restricted subject soundly as a part of Spanish history, Burke ranges far beyond the story of a single college of surgery. He touches with authority nearly every problem that marked the shift to modernism, not just in the professional college but in the Spanish universities as well—the "blood-purity" test for admission to institutions of higher learning (*limpieza de sangre*), censorship, the review of new surgical techniques, the trial-lecture of selecting professors, and the collapse of Latin as the language of medical education. Though he soundly fits all this into Spanish history, the answers he gets are not always what English and American education might prepare a reader for. Mention Spain in juxtaposition with censorship and such a man anywhere in the West outside the Iberian Peninsula is likely to conclude that he can make all the proper deductions from there out.

Yet censorship in the epoch of San Carlos, if it were a drama, would have a surprise ending. All the important new medical and surgical works from Great Britain, France, Holland, and Italy flowed in so freely that the process was not worth remarking. Spanish students of surgery could and did turn to Francois Quesnay, a Frenchman, on gangrene, to Benjamin Bell, a Scotsman, on tumors and ulcers, to Felix Fontana, an Italian, on wounds and poison complications, and to Percival Pott, an Irishman, on "contusions, dislocations, and fractures." They thus called to their support all "accredited authors" and, even in remote Guatemala, could boast that they had at their elbows the publications of the Royal Academy of Surgery and Medicine in Paris. The College in Madrid, in its capacity of adviser to the Council of Castile, did indirectly censor manuscripts in surgery, and to some degree in medicine, not to stifle learning and progress, but to prevent unscientific and dangerous work from imposing upon both the profession and the public. In a limited sense it also served the purpose of the modern medical journal. It heard and reviewed in open meeting the purported discoveries of its own professors as well as those of others, some from distant parts of the Empire, approved or rejected them outright, and recorded the findings. In the process of this work it disapproved a famous operation perfected by one of its own—Gimbernat's operation on the crural arch—and turned down Dr. Narcisco Esparragosa's "elastic forceps" as "not useful." This device combined obstetrical loops and filets or hafts made of whale bristles and was therefore impervious to the moisture that had rendered such loops useless since the time of Hippocrates and that had consequently encouraged the use of iron forceps, which appear to have been designed more for crushing and torture than for extricating a *criatura*, as the Spaniards so touchingly dubbed the infant. Although Dr. Burke is telling the story of a college and not writing the history of Spanish surgery, a thorough review of the records of these "discoveries" and procedures systematically presented by hopeful surgeons should give a very precise idea of what the average surgon then regarded as new. More and more the medical man began to turn up in the vanguard.

Despite the pompous Latin evasions put in the mouths of physicians and surgeons by eighteenth-century novelists, doctors generally were the first to expose the hypocrisy of conducting classes in stilted Latin and staging trial-lectures (*oposiciones*) in competition for professorships in the same language. When everybody knew that most students could understand Latin only in snatches and stereotypes, the continued use of the spoken language was a vainglorious performance for some professors and an ordeal for the others. Because the rules of the *oposición* required a man competing for a chair to keep on talking in the language of the Romans until the sand in the hourglass ran out, the most learned and highly respected professor sometimes had to sit down in abject humiliation while the sand was still trickling down. A few days later, when the still waters had restored his soul, he might write a letter of contrite apology. That San Carlos put an end to the hoary pretension that made such a crisis possible is a sure sign that the College was on its way to making surgery a more scientific and respected profession. However, the *oposición*, modified and expanded, but bereft of Latin, has continued in Spain to this day. Who can say, though, that it is not superior to the pathetic practice now evolving in this country, where every "committee of selection" with a piffling teaching job to fill alerts every new Ph.D. from Bangor to San Bernadino and sits for a few months in awesome judgment upon them.

Dr. Burke's work should give impetus to the writing of Spanish medical history by non-Spaniards, especially in the English language, not just to make the facts available to many more people, but to clarify and interpret for those whose knowledge is short and whose concerns are so different from those of Spaniards. After all, the writer must understand what his readers cannot be expected to know as well as he understands his documents. The translation of all the works of Spaniards on the medical history of their country—which of course is not possible—would not be enough. Besides, the objective foreign historian is the best defense against any charge or fear of national bias. Occasionally, too, as in this case, the foreign investigator may fill gaps in a way that would be useful even to Spaniards. The *protomedicato*, in which Spain was so clearly ahead of the rest of Europe in fixing the role of government in medicine, still clamors for its historian. Dr. Burke has clearly suggested that subjects such as this board of King's physicians would give non-Spanish authors precisely the kind of vehicle they need to write and interpret Spanish medical history outside the Peninsula without working over old ground.

JOHN TATE LANNING

*Durham, N. C.*
*December, 1975*

# Preface

The Royal College of San Carlos was established in Madrid in 1788 with the purpose of training surgeons. In the eyes of its founder, Antonio Gimbernat, however, this modest objective represented the culmination of years of efforts to reform Spanish surgery. Thus, the story of San Carlos is not only the story of a single institution, significant as that institution was, but the history of Spanish medical reform in the eighteenth century.

Spanish medicine has long been the exclusive concern of Spanish medical historians. Their contributions, in turn, have tended to concentrate on specific men, institutions, and disciplines to such an extent that a reader can easily conclude that medicine evolved in a political and social vacuum. Historians of the Spanish Enlightenment, on the other hand, have focused their attention on the more dramatic conflicts involving entrenched economic interests, new ideologies, and the Catholic Church. In truth, medical reform was intimately tied to the age in which it occurred, and the kind of reform represented by the College of San Carlos was the essence of Enlightenment in the eyes of the *ilustrados* themselves. It is the purpose of this study, then, to present the history of San Carlos in order to understand better the eighteenth-century reform of Spanish medicine, and to link that reform to the broader forces at work in eighteenth-century Spain itself.

The College of San Carlos was a landmark in Spanish medicine. Its founders carefully emulated the best of recent academic reform from Spain and abroad. As a result, a modern curriculum rooted in the natural sciences and based on contemporary authors, a thorough grounding in anatomy, and extensive clinical experience assured that surgeons who graduated from San Carlos were the equal of any in Europe. Yet the new college challenged the existing legal and social structure as well. Its success represented the transformation of surgery from a despised craft into a respectable profession, a veritable social revolution within medicine, and one that succeeded first in Spain. At the same time, its novel position under the direct patronage of the Crown signified the decline of autonomous university faculties and the rise of centralized, national education.

Just as the success of San Carlos was more than an intellectual victory, so, too, its opposition was rooted in more than blind adherence to tradition. Reform in surgical education inevitably threatened the traditional privileges of the universities and the Protomedicato, the social pretensions of university-trained physicians, and the traditional balance between royal power and professional autonomy. Further studies may well show that other reforms of the Spanish Enlightenment similarly entailed both intellectual and social issues.

In the study that follows, I have attempted to integrate the reform of medical education as exemplified by San Carlos with the broader issues of the Spanish Enlightenment. The first two chapters describe the objectives and institutions of reform, as well as the existing practices and structures of the medical profession. Chapter III examines the reform of medical education in universities and hospitals. The study then turns to San Carlos itself: the complex interplay of politics, ideas, and concerns of status that led to the creation of the college, the academic structures and accomplishments of the school, and its impact on medical education elsewhere in Spain. Unlike many Enlightenment studies, the story of San Carlos does not end in 1808, but continues through the tumultuous decades of invasion, reaction, and revolution that followed.

Many individuals have given generously of their time and talents during the course of this study. I am especially grateful to the late John Tate Lanning, who introduced me to the possibilities of examining eighteenth-century institutions of education and culture. Both personally and in his work he set forth the highest standards of scholarship and professionalism. His wise counsel, challenging suggestions, wealth of knowledge, demanding standards, and patience and encouragement, as well as his example, are in large part responsible for any merit this book possesses. Financial support for research in Spain was provided by the Hispanic Council of Duke University and the Consejo Superior de Investigaciones Científicas, where the gracious assistance of the capable staffs of the Spanish archives listed in the bibliography facilitated my research. Special mention is due the late Robert S. Smith, Miguel Bordonau, former director of the Biblioteca Nacional, and Remedios Migueles de Meudiluce of the Archivo de la Universidad Central. The studies on Spanish universities by George Addy and Richard Kagan were invaluable on that aspect of the story; Toby Gelfand provided constructive criticism based on his research on French surgery. The manuscript itself was no doubt improved as a result of the suggestions of Robert Durden, John Te Paske, James Bergquist and Linda K. Salvucci. Mrs. Bess Polkowski typed the manuscript with skill and patience. Villanova University generously subsidized the costs of publication. To all I am deeply grateful. Finally, my wife, Kathy deserves special thanks for her loving support and encouragement. I am alone responsible for any errors or shortcomings.

MICHAEL E. BURKE

*Villanova, Pa.*
*Dec. 1, 1976*

# THE ROYAL COLLEGE OF SAN CARLOS

CHAPTER I

# INTRODUCTION: THE ENLIGHTENMENT IN SPAIN

For some Spaniards the eighteenth century was a time of critical reexamination. Once endowed with military might, economic wealth, and prestigious universities, Spain had fallen into decline. The rest of Europe seemed to have passed her by. Indeed, "enlightened" foreigners now pointed to Spain and her colonies as the symbol of backwardness and decay. Such was the pessimistic view that characterized the Spanish Enlightenment.

Thus, it was possible to say, as it has been said, that Spain became more European during the eighteenth century than at any other period in her history. This arraignment is true, but it is so only because imitation seemed necessary in order to restore Spanish grandeur. Even so, the Spanish Enlightenment remained very Spanish.

The term "Enlightenment" frequently conjures up images of universal doubt and questioning, of demands that every belief and every institution be subjected to the critical examination of reason. As the new spirit of secularism, cosmopolitanism, and freedom captivated the new breed of intellectuals, the enlightened came to fear stagnation far more than they feared the unknown. The eighteenth century immediately brings to mind such philosophes as Voltaire and Rousseau with their impatient criticisms of society and their righteous secularism. Small wonder that historians have seldom used French medical schools as a means of describing the French Enlightenment.

The Enlightenment, however, involved more than political, social, and religious criticism. The optimism so characteristic of the eighteenth century also applied to the realm of knowledge. The remarkable discoveries in science seemed to suggest that man could achieve a complete understanding of the universe. He had the tools. He simply had to throw aside tradition and observe "how it works," be it the human body or the universe itself. Specific descriptions were not enough, however; eighteenth-century man had a penchant for discovering universal laws that explained everything. Since he assumed all nature was interdependent, he had to place all phenomena in a unified whole. Thus, one finds Carolus Linnaeus (1707–1778) developing a method of classifying all botanical life by a single system in his *Systema naturae*, and the Comte de Buffon (1707–1788) attempting to classify all nature in his *Histoire Naturelle*. No project was insurmountable. Governments—including that of Spain—and private academies and societies endeavored to collect specimens from all over the world. In 1759 the new Académie de Bordeaux embarked on a project to write a complete history of the earth.[1]

This eighteenth-century interest in compiling the findings of many observers led naturally to that modern tendency of scholars to organize academies and institutes dedicated to holding scholarly meetings, awarding prizes, and publishing journals. The English Royal Society had appeared in 1660; the French followed with the Académie des Sciences in 1662. Other societies devoted to specific sciences quickly followed. Most societies reflected the concern of the age with education, for only an enlightened public could properly exercise the freedom with which the eighteenth century was so preoccupied. Since the typical academy was convinced that ignorance was the principal barrier to progress, however, it endeavored not only to expand human knowledge but also to judge the accuracy of the assertions of others. Thus, the intellectuals of royal academies tended to become the arbiters of the new truth born of the scientific revolution. By its very nature, the academy was disinclined to encourage complete freedom for the circulation of ideas when so many popular beliefs seemed based on superstition and ignorance. Royal patronage increased the dominant position of the academy, which, in turn, gave monarchs a significant influence in national intellectual life.[2]

Yet the Enlightenment, including its scientific aspects, was essentially an international movement. Books and periodicals spread the new knowledge among scholars and the public at large without regard for

1. Paul Hazard, *European Thought in the Eighteenth Century from Montesquieu to Lessing*, trans. J. Lewis May (Cleveland, 1963), p. 135. For further discussion of the Enlightenment and science, see Peter Gay, *The Enlightenment: An Interpretation* (2 vols.; New York, 1966, 1969); George Rudé, *Europe in the Eighteenth Century* (New York, 1973); Herbert Butterfield, *The Origins of Modern Science* (2nd ed., rev.; New York, 1957); Ernst Cassirer, *The Philosophy of the Enlightenment*, trans. Fritz C. A. Koelin and James P. Pettegrove (Princeton, 1961); A. Wolf, *A History of Science, Technology, and Philosophy in the Eighteenth Century* (New York, 1939).

2. On the French Academy, see Roger Hahn, *The Anatomy of Scientific Institutions: The Paris Academy of Sciences, 1666–1803* (Berkeley, 1971), esp. pp. 7–60.

national boundaries. Scientists became international figures. The medical educator, Gerard Van Swieten (1700–1772), for example, studied medicine at Leyden and went on to supervise medical education at the University of Vienna. Meanwhile, most of Western Europe used his textbook.[3] The hope was that the application of new knowledge would improve all aspects of human life throughout the civilized world.

In Spain the Enlightenment centered primarily upon this scientific purpose. Unlike many French philosophes, the Spanish *ilustrado* was immensely practical. He saw the new sciences not as the key to all truth but as concrete tools to improve human life. Again and again, the Spanish innovators used the term "useful knowledge." Their reaction to the rigid abstractions of the still prevalent scholasticism quite naturally led them to prefer practical applications to universal theories. Thus, the Spanish Enlightenment reflected the utilitarian thrust of the later Enlightenment throughout Europe, but it largely ignored the more idealistic concerns with rationalism and natural law that also characterized that intellectual movement elsewhere in Europe.[4]

The fear if not the realization that Spain had declined provided the greatest incentive toward reform. The feeling that somewhere something was very wrong permeated the century. Years of inaction had left Spain in many respects underdeveloped compared with other European nations. Old customs and values remained that had outlived their usefulness. Many advocates of reform, for example, expressed concern at the disdain with which most Spaniards looked upon commerce and industry. Joseph Moñino, one of the most enlightened ministers of Charles III, noted that progress was to be found primarily in undoing accumulated wrongs.[5] One had to remove the obstacles to progress. At the same time the ilustrados were very conscious of themselves as something new and different, as "muy siglo XVIII." They were imbued with a strong sense of mission to correct the accumulated wrongs, from decadent universities and feudal landholdings to an all-powerful Church and one of the largest beggar classes in Europe. Pro-

3. *Commentaria in H. B.* (Herman Boerhaave) *Aphorismos de cognoscendis et curandis morbus*. See Arturo Castiglioni, *A History of Medicine*, trans. E. B. Krumbhaar (New York, 1941), pp. 617–618.

4. On this distinction, see Gay, *The Enlightenment*, II. esp. 459; and Arthur P. Whitaker, "Changing and Unchanging Interpretations of the Enlightenment in Spanish America," *Proceedings of the American Philosophical Society*, CXIV (Aug. 1970), 263.

5. Pedro Voltes, *Carlos III y su tiempo* (Barcelona, 1964), p. 10. On this theme, see also Luis Sánchez Agesta, *El pensamiento político del despotismo ilustrado* (Madrid, 1953), pp. 13–18; Antonio Domínguez Ortiz, *La sociedad española en el siglo XVIII* (Madrid, 1955), pp. 40 ff., 393–394; William J. Callahan, *Honor, Commerce, and Industry in Eighteenth-Century Spain* (Boston, 1972).

pagandists wrote not just for the king but for an increasingly disturbed public.[6]

Even before 1700, of course, Spaniards were not completely immersed in ignorance. In 1692, for example, a minor cleric, Juan Cruzade de la Cruz, possessed a library of more than 1,125 volumes including Francis Bacon and Descartes.[7] During the first half of the eighteenth century numerous writers pointed out the problems facing Spain. Although they were men of words, not of action, their impact in alerting future generations to the need for major reforms was substantial.

Later generations endeavored to create institutional support for their ideas by establishing societies and academies similar to those abroad. Public and private efforts cooperated to establish the National Library (1711), the Spanish Academy (1713), the Academy of History (1735), and such scientific institutes as the Botanical Garden and a museum of natural history. Prominent among private efforts were the Economic Societies for Friends of the Country that appeared in many Spanish and Spanish-American cities. These societies set out to encourage better methods in agriculture and industry. They sponsored lectures, published research, and, in some cases, even established schools.[8]

Spanish reformers were not radical men, at least not in the usual sense of the word. Most were loyal Spaniards who did not challenge authority. No major institutions except for the Society of Jesus were suppressed. These reformers realized, however, that Spain needed a change in outlook above all else. This most fundamental change of all is what Spanish reformers attempted. The Spanish mind was to be brought up to date. Benito Jerónimo Feijóo (1676–1764), the Benedictine monk who more than any other individual tried to change Spanish attitudes, constantly emphasized this theme. Spanish schools were backward in science, he wrote, because Spaniards looked upon new discoveries as "useless curiosities."[9] Intellectuals had to lose their suspicion of anything novel and stop pretending that what they did not know was not worth knowing.[10] In other words, Spaniards would have to

6. José Munoz Pérez, "La España de Carlos III y su conciencia de período histórico," in Manuel Fernández Alvarez (ed.), *Estudios sobre historia de España* (Madrid, 1965), pp. 358 ff.; Sánchez Agesta, *El pensamiento político*, pp. 87–88.

7. Henry Kamen, *The Spanish Inquisition* (New York, 1965), p. 252.

8. On the Economic Societies, see Robert Jones Shafer, *The Economic Societies in the Spanish World* (Syracuse, N.Y., 1958); Ignacio María Barriola, *Los Amigos del País y la medicina* (San Sebastián, 1963).

9. Benito Jerónimo Feijóo y Montenegro, *Cartas eruditas, y curiosas* (2nd ed.; Madrid, 1781), tom. III, núm. 34, pp. 452 ff.

10. *Ibid.*, tom. II, núm. 16, pp. 246–247.

learn to accept different standards in order for Spain to prosper. Reason and experience were the proper criteria of truth. Man has never made progress when his reason was divorced from experience.[11] This great eclectic modernizer was thus most Spanish in avoiding the excessive formulation of universal laws.

Other reformers agreed that a change in values was a fundamental prerequisite to institutional reform, even in economic matters. At the root of economic backwardness, they argued, was the popular scorn for manual labor, a prejudice that encouraged some to rely on charity rather than to work with their hands. Instead of advocating a complete break with the past, however, these reformers urged that honor, that traditional incentive in Spanish society, be bestowed on the mechancal arts as well.[12]

Such moderate reformers as Feijóo should not be associated with propagandists of the Black Legend. They did not believe that Spain was inherently backward. Indeed, Feijóo suggested that the pedantry that had captured higher education was not at all typical. The revival of true science would be more in keeping with Spanish tradition.[13]

Of course, foreign ideas also had considerable influence on Spanish reformers, an aspect of the Enlightenment that has provoked considerable debate among historians. Jean Sarrailh suggests that Spanish progress was proportional to the reception given to foreigners and their suggestions.[14] Certainly, many of the academies founded during the century were built upon foreign models. Yet enlightened Spaniards were very selective in choosing the ideas they would import, and, in doing so, they imprinted their own preoccupation with "useful science" and practical change. As a result, the Enlightenment in Spain was not a pale imitation of that movement elsewhere but a careful adaptation of knowledge from abroad chosen to provide practical solutions for Spanish problems.

A good example of foreign influence in the "useful sciences" may be found in the field of mining. In 1752 a young Spanish mathematician studying in Paris encouraged William Bowles, an English chemist, to return with him to Almadén, the important mercury mine. Bowles

11. Feijóo, *Teatro crítico*, tom. I, disc. 5 and tom. V, disc. 11, in *Obras escogidas*, ed. Agustín Millares Carlo (4 vols.; "Biblioteca de Autores Españoles," vols. 56 [Madrid, 1863], and 141–153 [Madrid, 1961]), II, 51, and III, 237, respectively.

12. Callahan, *Honor, Commerce, and Industry*, pp. 46–47.

13. This distinction is developed in Sánchez Agesta, *El pensamiento político*, pp. 74 ff.

14. Jean Sarrailh, *La España ilustrada de la segunda mitad del siglo XVIII*, trans. Antonio Alatorre (Mexico City, 1957).

agreed, and while he was there he set up a modern chemistry laboratory and instituted several mining reforms. Word of the spirit of innovation that existed at Almadén spread. German engineers, encouraged by attractive salaries, arrived in considerable numbers and gave instructions to young Spaniards. In 1777 Charles III, who was eagerly watching these developments, formally established a Royal School of Subterranean Geometry and Mineralogy.

Meanwhile, the Spanish navy was searching for better methods and materials to make heavy guns. In 1770 it paid two recent graduates of the informal Almadén school to journey through the major cities of Europe to learn all that they could about mining. One of the two, Fausto Elhuyar, studied under Abraham Werner, the most prominent German geologist of the day. Elhuyar returned to offer classes at the newly established school at Almadén, and later he journeyed to New Spain to promote a school of mining there.[15] Thus, in a few decades, the most advanced mining techniques were known and used in Spain and the Empire.

This type of cooperative effort by private citizens and government to make modern technology available in Spain was typical of foreign influence there. Most Spaniards who went abroad returned as skilled technicians, not as political radicals. (Of course, scientists crossed national boundaries frequently in the eighteenth century; Spain was not unique.) Indeed, Spain sought foreign skills and techniques far more than foreign philosophies and ideologies. Carolus Linnaeus, the botanist, and Hermann Boerhaave (1668–1738), a prominent medical educator, may have been more important to enlightened Spaniards than Diderot or Rousseau. Spaniards borrowed the emphasis on observation and usefulness, not the pure rationalism of Descartes or the anticlericalism of Voltaire. Most Spanish reformers saw little merit in open rebellion or violent change.

Given the pragmatic concerns of Spanish reformers, English sources probably had more influence than French ones. Spaniards could readily identify with a nation that, at once, valued its own traditions, yet was open to new ideas.[16] Feijóo, for example, was probably most greatly influenced by Francis Bacon and by his fellow Spaniard, Pedro Martín

15. Arthur P. Whitaker, "The Elhuyar Mining Mission and the Enlightenment," *Hispanic American Historical Review*, XXXI (1951), 556–585; Clement G. Motten, *Mexican Silver and the Enlightenment* (Philadelphia, 1950), pp. 6–7.

16. John H. R. Polt, *Jovellanos and His English Sources* (Philadelphia, 1965); Whitaker, "The Elhuyar Mining Mission," p. 263.

Martínez (1684–1736).[17] More typical, still, were the numerous teachers, writers, and even clerics throughout the Peninsula who did what they could to spread practical knowledge and improve the lot of their countrymen. The Salamancan professor who introduced new texts or the bishop who joined a local society to improve the economy did not necessarily think of himself as a Francophile.[18]

Perhaps the attitude toward religion best exemplifies this selective approach to foreign ideas. Most ilustrados carefully distinguished between religion's potentially stifling effect on science and religion itself, and between superstition and excessive Church wealth and Spain's Catholic heritage. The secularism of the Spanish Enlightenment wanted to restore religious belief to its proper place, not to eliminate it from national life. Feijóo repeatedly emphasized that experimental science was not a threat to Catholicism. Charles III, who expelled the Jesuits and set up numerous secular schools, attended daily Mass and devoted long hours to his personal spiritual life.[19]

But in spite of their moderation, the ilustrados represented only a small part of the Spanish people. The division of eighteenth-century Spain was not one between French ideas on the one hand and the Inquisition on the other. Rather, it was between a small number of middle- and upper-class reformers and a proud, conservative, even complacent people. Most members of the aristocracy continued to think more of prestige than of political power. Spaniards in the main were indifferent to reform and a little suspicious of anything foreign. Many felt the new spirit was somehow alien and "un-Spanish," perhaps a threat to Spain's role as the supposed bastion of orthodox Catholicism.

Thus, the Spanish Enlightenment sprang from a small number of Spaniards. That they had some success was due to the happy fact that the Bourbon monarchs, especially Charles III, appointed forward-looking Spaniards to critical positions. The power of the Crown enabled the ilustrados to put their ideas into effect.

17. Gregorio Marañón, "Las ideas biológicas del P. Feijóo, in Feijóo, *Obras escogidas*, II, xxxii–lx. Pedro Martín Martínez was a bitter critic of the state of Spanish medicine. He revived public anatomical demonstrations at the Hospital General of Madrid and wrote numerous medical tracts.

18. On foreign influence, see Sarrailh, *La España ilustrada*, pp. 111–140; Muñoz Pérez, "La España de Carlos III," pp. 364–365; Richard Herr, *The Eighteenth-Century Revolution in Spain* (Princeton, 1958), pp. 31 ff.; Juan Reglá Campistol and Santiago Alcolea, *El siglo XVIII* (Barcelona, 1959), p. 43; Shafer, *The Economic Societies*, pp. 24 ff.

19. Vicente Rodríguez Casado, "Iglesia y estado en el reinado de Carlos III," *Estudios americanos*, I (1948), 7–25; Sánchez Agesta, *El pensamiento político*, pp. 166 ff.

The relationship between the ilustrados and the Crown is essential in explaining the reforms of eighteenth-century Spain, for, to some degree, each at the same time agreed with the other and used the other. While reformers looked upon traditional institutions as bastions of closed-mindedness, the Crown also viewed them as barriers to increasing royal power. Thus, reformers and royal officials worked hand in hand in the creation of new institutions that would both promote modern ideas and limit the autonomy of traditional bodies. As a result, reform in Spain was virtually synonomous with the growth of royal influence, particularly in education and the learned professions.

The close relationship between reform and the attack on ancient privileges, or *fueros*, also helps to account for the small number of Spaniards who actively opposed the increasing political influence of the reformers. Men such as the powerful Duke of Alba, for example, who bitterly opposed the appointment of the liberal Conde de Aranda as president of the Council of Castile,[20] was probably as concerned with the growth of royal power as with the intellectual reform he represented. For with reform, traditional fueros came into question. Since even all the new academies of science were under royal control, they threatened the traditional, autonomous authority of universities, guilds, and courts of special jurisdiction. As such, they probably aroused the universal antipathy of a new, meddlesome bureaucracy as well.

In light of the crucial role of the Crown in eighteenth-century reforms, therefore, it is as important to understand the objectives and viewpoints of royal officials as it is to understand the ilustrados themselves. When the Bourbon family came to the throne of Spain in 1700, Spain once again had monarchs who, to say the least, were interested in Spain's future. The first two monarchs, Philip V (1700–1746) and Ferdinand VI (1746–1759), approached the nation's problems with programs similar to those of the Catholic monarchs two hundred years before. Once again Spain was governed as a nation, not as a dynasty with unclear foreign dimensions. In order for Spain to recover her prestige abroad, she first had to concentrate on domestic development. Centralization of power would secure the position of the monarch. Economic reforms would increase national prosperity and power.

In 1714 Aragón-Catalonia lost her autonomy as punishment for supporting the Hapsburgs in the War of Spanish Succession. Henceforth, Spain would have one Cortes and one language. Catalan universities

20. Vicente Rodríguez Casado, *La política y los políticos en el reinado de Carlos III* (Madrid, 1962), p. 151.

were suppressed and the University of Cervera established to bring Catalans into Castilian life. This final union had the unforeseen effect of encouraging Catalans to find opportunities in Castile. A substantial number of the supporters of the surgical colleges in Castile would come from Catalonia.

Steps taken by Philip and Ferdinand to improve Spain's economic position no doubt encouraged the proponents of reform. The two monarchs built roads and canals, reformed tax collection, and restricted the *mesta*, or sheepherders' guild. Though most of their chief ministers were not Spanish, both monarchs were eager to assist Spanish reformers. In 1748 a group of naval surgeons persuaded Ferdinand VI to establish the first Royal School of Surgery at Cádiz.

The greatest support these monarchs gave Spanish reformers, though, was in establishing the tradition and machinery of a central government for all Spain. Philip V streamlined the operation of the Royal and Supreme Council of Castile, first established in the fourteenth century, and gave it final authority in all domestic questions. This Council would become the principal government agent of reform. During the eighteenth century the Council had twenty-two councilors, most of whom held other important posts simultaneously. The president of the Council ranked just under the king in social prestige. Probably even more influential than the councilors were the three *fiscals* (two for Castile, one for Aragón). The *fiscals*, or crown attorneys, wrote reports, provided information, and in general prepared the business of the Council. All public education, including the universities and schools of religious orders, fell under the jurisdiction of the Council of Castile.[21]

The greatest achievements of Spain's reformers occurred during the reign of Charles III (1759–1788). The new monarch intended to restore Spain's greatness by using his royal powers to the fullest. Like his predecessors, he brought many foreigners to Spain with him as advisers, but the Esquilache revolts of 1766 made him painfully aware that he could not force modernization upon Spain by decree.[22] As a result, he decided to name Spaniards to strategic positions.

Charles, no intellectual himself, always paid close attention to his

21. *Novísima recopilación de las leyes de España* (3 vols.; Madrid, 1805), lib. IV, tit. iii, ley 4, and lib. IV, tit, xvi, ley 5 (hereinafter cited as *Nov. rec.*, IV, iii, 4); Georges Desdevises du Dezert, "Les institutions de l'Espagne au XVIIIe siècle," *Revue Hispanique*, LXX (1927), 67–93.

22. In 1766 Charles III's Italian minister, Esquilache, ordered the people of Madrid to wear French-style short coats and tricorns. Outraged Madrileños, already angry at the number of foreigners in government, rose up in fury, forcing the king to flee to Aranjuez.

advisers. Thus, his choices were critical. Much of the progress of his reign was due to the men he chose to assist him. Indeed, both supporters and critics of his reign agree that his ministers were responsible for most of its accomplishments.[23] Three of these men, the Conde de Aranda, the Conde de Floridablanca (José Moñino), and the Conde de Campomanes, played especially important roles in educational reforms.

One historian dubbed the Conde de Aranda (1719–1798) the real governor of Spain between 1766 and 1773, for, as president of the Council of Castile, all major internal reforms passed through his hands.[24] Aranda was a man of contradictions. From a wealthy Aragón family, he often sympathized with the Church and the nobility and looked down upon the lower classes; yet he was an intense Francophile and preferred to walk through the streets of Madrid rather than ride in a luxurious coach. One of his first acts was to set up public entertainments in Madrid. Little wonder that the aristocracy disliked him. He had been educated abroad, was an acquaintance of Voltaire, and had served in the army and diplomatic corps before coming to Madrid. Known for his progressive outlook, he was nevertheless more a man of action than an intellectual.[25]

Second in influence were the two fiscals, José Moñino (1728–1808) and the Conde de Campomanes (1723–1803). Unlike Aranda, neither came from the upper nobility. During their university careers both had been *manteistas*, that is, they had been shut out of the prestigious *colegios mayores*. Both Moñino and Campomanes were noted liberals, and neither hesitated to attack the traditional privileges of powerful institutions.[26]

José Moñino, later the Count of Floridablanca, was fiscal until 1772, when he became minister of state. He played a key role in the expulsion

23. For example, Sarrailh, *La España illustrada*, pp. 122 ff.; Marcelino Menéndez y Pelayo, *Historia de los heterodoxos españoles* ("Obras completas," vols. 35–42; Madrid, 1940–1959), XXXIX, 17 (Menéndez y Pelayo pointedly blames Charles's ministers, not Charles, for "la impiedad francesa."); Domínguez Ortiz, *La sociedad española*, pp. 33–40; Cayetano Alcázar Molina, "El despotismo ilustrado en España," *Bulletin of the International Committee of Historical Sciences*, V (1933), 728–731; Voltes, *Carlos III*, pp. 17–20; Antonio Ballesteros y Beretta, *Historia de España y su influencia en la historia universal* (10 vols., 2nd ed., rev.; Madrid, 1958), IX, 13–22.

24. Alcázar Molina, "El despotismo ilustrado," V, 731.

25. Francisco Espinosa y González Pérez, "El Conde de Aranda," *La España Moderna*, XXI (1909), 5–18; Rodríguez Casado, *La política . . . de Carlos III*, pp. 205–217; Desdevises du Dezert, "Les institutions," pp. 41–44.

26. For Moñino and Campomanes, see Desdevises du Dezert, "Les institutions," pp. 44–48; Rodríguez Casado, *La política . . . de Carlos III*, pp. 227–229; Reglá Campistol, *El siglo XVIII*, pp. 84–85

of the Jesuits and in winning government support for the Economic Societies.

Pedro Rodríguez, the Conde de Campomanes, was the intellectual of the Council. Few men exercised the position of fiscal to such telling effect. As both a perceptive writer and realistic statesman, Campomanes set out to reform Spain by destroying the autonomy of the many privileged institutions, including the universities and the guilds. His two major works, *Discurso sobre el fomento de la industria popular* (*Discourse on the Development of Popular Industry*) and *Discurso sobre la educación de los artesanos y su fomento* (*Discourse on the Education of Artisans and Its Development*), were classics in their perceptive analyses of Spain's economic problems.

Campomanes believed that government had the obligation to promote the general welfare of all subjects. Thus, an institution was harmful if it benefited only a few at the expense of the many, or if its autonomy from government was so extensive that it prevented effective royal action in a particular area. Only privilege that improved the public good was tolerable. Convinced that economic development was essential, he judged educational reforms in light of their practical potential.[27]

In 1773 Charles III sent Aranda abroad and replaced him with Manuel Ventura Figueroa. Described by one historian as "a venal, intriguing cleric,"[28] the new president of the Council of Castile had little sympathy with the reformers. The pace of change became slower. Ten years later, however, Campomanes became president of the Council, and the reformers were once again in charge.

Most of the new schools and academies that so characterized the emphasis on "useful knowledge" of the Spanish Enlightenment were therefore the result of a combination of private initiative and government support.[29] The government of Charles III was intensely interested in educational reform, both to promote "useful knowledge" so as to support economic development, and to remold public attitudes. To be sure, the Bourbon monarchs did not introduce enlightened thought to Spain, but they and their ministers did provide essential financial, legal,

27. On Campomanes's thought, see Ricardo Krebs Wilckens, *El pensamiento histórico, político y económico del Conde de Campomanes* (Santiago, Chile, 1960); Felipe Alvarez Requejo, *El Conde de Campomanes: Su obra historica* (Oviedo, 1954).

28. Rodríguez Casado, *La política . . . de Carlos III*, p. 226.

29. In addition to the surgical colleges, schools of pharmacy, astronomy, mineralogy, and navigation apparently came about in this manner.

and moral support to indigenous reformers. Indeed, it was the Crown that enabled a minority of liberals to establish the institutions needed to propagate their ideas.

The Crown also acted frequently on its own initiative. Campomanes, for example, had precipitated the establishment of all but three of the sixty-eight Economic Societies for Friends of the Country that existed by 1791. The Crown erected new colleges and patronized public lectures, invited foreigners to visit Spain, and provided scholarships for Spaniards to study abroad. The government of Charles III also embarked on vast public works projects, attempted to colonize unused land, founded the Bank of San Carlos, and liberalized trade with America. No doubt its most dramatic action was the expulsion of the Jesuits from Spain in 1767. Since the departure of these teachers gave the Crown the opportunity to set up its own brand of education in the confiscated schools, the expulsion of the Jesuits inadvertently marked the beginning of extensive royal participation in educational reform and intervention in previously self-governing schools and universities. The former Jesuit Imperial College of Madrid reopened as the Royal Studies of San Isidro in 1771 with a thoroughly revised curriculum. Courses included mathematics, physics, and natural law. In other efforts to reform education, the Crown established free elementary and trade schools, dictated minimum standards for teachers, and undertook a major reform of the nation's universities.

Charles III also devoted considerable attention to improving Madrid, a city of some 200,000 inhabitants. He transformed his capital from a squalid, dirty town into a modern city with wide brightly lighted boulevards, imposing monuments, and magnificent public buildings. In numerous decrees he attempted to eliminate the ubiquitous beggars and to improve sanitary conditions. New roads radiated out from Madrid. He even placed charitable institutions under a Royal General Board of Welfare (*Real Junta General de Caridad*) to allocate funds to hospitals and poorhouses.[30] Thus, it was not surprising that Charles was receptive to proposals to include better medical care in his model city.

In sum, the Crown had two objectives during the eighteenth century: to increase royal power at the expense of traditional, autonomous institutions; and to support Spanish reformers as long as they did not

30. Charles E. Kany, *Life and Manners in Madrid, 1750–1800* (Berkeley, 1932); Enrique de Tapia Ozcariz, *Carlos III y su época* (Madrid, 1962), p. 370; José Alvarez-Sierra, *Carlos III y la higiene pública* (Madrid, 1956).

threaten royal prerogatives. Thus, in the realm of science and "useful knowledge," the interests of the reformers and the Crown were identical, so significant progress occurred.

The efforts of the Spanish reformers during the reign of Charles III can be easily dismissed with the phrase "too little, too late," but, in fact, the fault was not in the plans and ideas. Most of the "original" ideas, from more laboratory science to a less powerful Church, had been suggested before, but Spain's shortcomings had been more political than intellectual. The significance of Charles III, then, was less in his goals than in his eagerness to put some of these new ideas into action.

The ilustrados failed to destroy what they themselves believed were the principal stumbling blocks to progress. The Inquisition endured to the point of successfully prosecuting Pablo de Olavide, the liberal accomplice of Campomanes who directed the reform of the University of Seville. The all-powerful mesta and the acres and acres of land held as a *mayorazgo* (entailed estate) remained. Worst of all was the concept of *limpieza de sangre* (purity of blood), which restricted the educational and employment opportunities, by custom when not rigidly enforced, of a man who was tainted by the Inquisition or by non-Catholic ancestors. And most of the Spanish people remained poor and ignorant as before.

Yet, in another sense, the reformers were a success. If they sometimes placed too much faith in laws and institutions, they were nevertheless far too realistic to believe they could transform Spain overnight, and too practical to be captivated by visions of a utopia. Their goal was not immediate social revolution but reform directed from above. By reforming the education of a few, they hoped that a new mentality would slowly trickle down to the many in succeeding generations. Thus, it was natural that both education and medicine became significant focal points of the Spanish Enlightenment; an institution dedicated to the improvement of surgical training, such as the Royal College of San Carlos, represented the very essence of enlightened objectives. Surgical training that was concerned with the "How?" and not the "Why?" was precisely the kind of "useful knowledge" that concerned progressive Spaniards. A brief examination of the importance of education and medicine will demonstrate this further.

Since Spanish backwardness was caused by outmoded manners of thought, reformers naturally devoted much attention to education. Many schools were archaic and excessively formalistic. Primary education was concerned with little more than Latin grammar. University learning was by rote. Nowhere were students encouraged to rely on observation and experience.

The ultimate objective of many educational reformers was to promote economic development. The importance of modern science was its potential usefulness in improving everyday life. The "useful sciences" were emphasized; students were to be taught what they could put to use. Feijóo even argued that the philosophy required of all medical students should be eliminated.[31] Gaspar Melchor de Jovellanos (1744–1811), the economist who served as adviser to several monarchs, complained that Spain had too many doctors, lawyers, and theologians, but not enough practical technicians to solve practical problems. He believed that if technical skills were held in higher esteem, more men would acquire them.[32] Indeed, one of the fundamental goals of the Spanish Enlightenment was to eliminate the widespread ignorance and superstition among the common folk. The nation had to be educated in practical, productive skills in order for Spain to realize her great economic potential. Thus, a new school was just as valuable as a new mine or a new factory. On the other hand, the royal ministers had no desire to create the questioning, cynical mind associated with the French Enlightenment. Education would still consist of transmitting facts, but the facts would be useful ones.[33]

This paradoxical attitude in education was even apparent in censorship policies. During the 1760s the Council of Castile prohibited the circulation of the works of Jesuit philosophers, including Francisco Suárez, in an effort to end the Jansenist controversy. But when the Inquisition placed the French *Encyclopédie* on the Index, Campomanes ordered that the articles on arts and crafts be published separately, purged of their offensive passages.[34] There was no disposition to bar scientific work from abroad.

Since medicine was the traditional profession most associated with the natural sciences, the glaring weaknesses in medical training and practice represented the shortcomings of Spanish science in general.

31. Feijóo, *Teatro crítico*, tom. VII, disc. 14, in *Obras*, III, 469–470.

32. Sánchez Agesta, *El pensamiento político*, pp. 125–49.

33. *Ibid.*, pp. 89, 195–200; Sarrailh, *La España ilustrada, pp.* 155–186.

34. Kamen, *The Spanish Inquisition*, pp. 257 ff.; Herr, *The Eighteenth-Century Revolution*, p. 43; Sánchez Agesta, *El pensamiento político*, pp. 109–13. During the eighteenth century the Council of Castile asserted its own right to censor publications. After 1768 the Council had the final voice in all censorship cases.

Feijóo's writings contain countless references to the backward state of the art. The preoccupation with medicine was also indicative of the pragmatism of the Enlightenment in Spain as it was elsewhere, for improvements in medical care and public health were highly visible and of obvious benefit. Moreover, any potential threat of medicine to political and religious orthodoxy was remote.

Medical education had never been as obscurantist as other disciplines, if only because it inherently required some contact with nature. The medical faculty at the University of Valencia, which was relatively progressive throughout the seventeenth century, was the source of substantial criticism of traditional medicine in the decades before 1700.[35] In 1697, physicians in Seville formed a medical society to supplement the backwardness of medical education in the university.[36] The Seville society was one of the first scientific academies devoted to the advancement of learning. During the eighteenth century three ilustrados concerned with medicine deserve special mention: Feijóo, Pedro Martín Martínez, and Andrés Piquer.

Benito Feijóo was the dominant figure in attacking the status quo. He attributed much of Spain's backwardness to her disdain for science. Observation and experience, he wrote, must replace the reliance upon ancient authorities. A prudent lack of confidence in traditional methods would be healthy. In his prolific writings he repeatedly attacked the backward state of Spanish universities. He recognized the need for anatomy in medical education, though he lacked such training himself. Feijóo also deplored the excessive concern for feminine modesty that often prevented obstetrical patients from receiving adequate care, since only women practiced that art even though men were usually better trained.

Pedro Martín Martínez, a close friend of Feijóo, also recognized the need for anatomy. In *Noches anatómicas* he bitterly disclosed how one could be licensed in medicine without ever dissecting a cadaver. To remedy this, he set up an anatomical theater in Madrid in 1705, in

35. José María López Piñero, "Harvey's Doctrine of the Blood in Seventeenth-Century Spain," *Journal of the History of Medicine and Allied Sciences*, XXVIII (1973), 230–242.

36. Gaspar Melchor de Jovellanos, *Informe dió como juez subdelegado del Real Protomedicato en Sevilla . . . sobre el estado de la Sociedad Médica de aquella ciudad, y del estudio de medicina en su universidad*, in *Obras . . . de Jovellanos*, ed. Candido Nocedal (2 vols.; "Biblioteca de Autores Españoles," vols. 46, 50 [Madrid, 1858]) I, 279–283. Hereinafter cited as Jovellanos, *Informe, . . . sobre medicina*, all of which is in Vol. I. The Seville society is discussed further in Chapter II.

which he offered dissections for the public. Though his own writings on anatomy contained many errors, he was instrumental in restoring anatomy to medical training.[37]

Andrés Piquer (1711–1772), who taught anatomy at the progressive University of Valencia, was better known for his experimental approach, his wide knowledge, and his written works than for his specific discoveries. His *Física moderna, racional y experimental* was the first Spanish text to argue that physics should be completely separate from philosophy since it can proceed only from empirical evidence. Though he apparently never dissected a cadaver, he instilled in a generation of students the need for patient clinical observation.[38] Anatomy and clinical training would form the basis of the new medical schools.

Throughout the eighteenth century medical progress continued as a result of the activities of individual doctors. In 1734 Feijóo was instrumental in founding the Madrid Academy of Medicine and Surgery, which was designed in imitation of similar scientific academies in Spain and abroad. In the academy, Feijóo hoped, scholars could pursue unrestricted study and research. The Madrid academy also published the *Efemérides Barométrico-médicas Matritenses*, the first Spanish monthly devoted exclusively to science, in order to circulate new discoveries from abroad.[39] Other less learned men, too, were eager to learn as much as possible. In 1716 a young barber-surgeon from Tarragona, Pedro Virgili, was so interested in anatomy that he journeyed to Montpellier to learn more.[40] He would return to establish the first Spanish college of surgery in Cádiz.

Whether a gradual transformation of government, education, and the professions was capable of bringing about basic changes in Spanish society remains doubtful. Effective moderate reform requires flexibility from established institutions and a spirit of consensus on the part of the public. Hindsight tells us Spain apparently had neither. In any event, the French invasion and the reaction that followed deprived Spanish ilustrados of the opportunity to taste the fruits of their efforts.

37. Eduardo García del Real, *Historia de la medicina en España* (Madrid, 1921), 418–422; Marañón, "Las ideas biológicas," pp. lxvii ff.

38. Sarrailh, *La España ilustrada*, pp. 423–424. Piquer's *Instituciones médicas* was used as a text at Montpellier.

39. Marañón, "Las ideas biológicas," pp. cxi, cxli; Henry F. Schulte, *The Spanish Press, 1470–1966: Print, Power and Politics* (Urbana, Ill., 1968), p. 87.

40. Diego Ferrer, *Historia del Real Colegio de Cirugía de la Armada de Cádiz* (Cádiz, 1961), p. 5. Hereinafter cited as Ferrer, *Colegio de Cádiz*.

CHAPTER II

# SPANISH MEDICINE IN THE EIGHTEENTH CENTURY

MEDICINE, one of man's oldest professions, did not become a science until modern times. To be sure, every society has felt the need for someone to heal the wounds and treat the diseases of its members, but it took many centuries for men of medicine to develop effective cures, and at least as long for the public to acquire confidence in its medical practitioners. By necessity, every society has felt greater need to regulate its doctors than to interfere with its scientists or artists. The man of medicine tampers not only with human life and comfort but also with the most basic moral principles of the men and society he serves.

Though the primary objective of the Royal College of Surgery of Madrid was to train surgeons, far more was involved. Was surgery a profession? What was its relationship to internal medicine? Would new methods and theories imply that accepted ones were erroneous? How should the opposing concepts of doctor as scientist and doctor as skilled craftsman be reconciled? Should the school that granted degrees also regulate the profession? Was medicine better regulated by men of medicine or by the state? In order to better understand the implications of these and other questions, it is necessary to examine the state of Spanish medicine in the eighteenth century.

For centuries Spanish men of medicine had been among the best in Europe. When the Moslems occupied Spain they established numerous teaching hospitals, made substantial advances in pharmacology, and initiated state regulation of doctors. The encyclopedic writings of Avicenna (980–1037), for example, carried on the traditions of Greek medicine and provided specific descriptions of diseases and cures.[1]

1. References to the history of medicine in general are primarily based on Fielding H. Garrison, *An Introduction to the History of Medicine* (4th ed., rev.; Philadelphia, 1929); Castiglioni, *A History of Medicine*; Charles Singer and E. Ashwood Underwood, *A Short History of Medicine* (New York, 1962); Richard A. Leonardo, *History of Surgery* (New York, 1943); Theodor Puschmann, *A History of Medical Education*,

During the Reconquest, Spaniards were quick to assimilate the knowledge accumulated by the Moslems. The Royal Ordinances of the University of Salamanca, prepared under Alfonso X (*el Sabio*) in 1254, seem to have provided for medical instruction.[2] Unfortunately, the statutes also provided for lower salaries for medical professors than for those in law, thereby suggesting that medicine was a less desirable profession. In any event, by the fourteenth century medicine was one of the major university faculties, and the universities had established themselves as the principal institutions engaged in medical education. Classroom medicine consisted primarily of learning the classic works of Hippocrates and Galen, both of whom remained the essence of medical education until the eighteenth century.[3]

For Hippocrates and Galen, the human body was best understood within a broad philosophy of human nature.[4] Hippocrates believed that health was the harmonious functioning of the four humors, or bodily fluids (blood, phlegm, yellow bile, and black bile), and the other organs of the body, that is, when the body was in a state of equilibrium. Illness was the result of an imbalance that the physician must correct. Centuries later, Galen (A.D. 129–199) synthesized Hippocratic medicine, Aristotelian philosophy, his experience dissecting animals, and a healthy dose of logic into a systematic, all-inclusive explanation of the human body. For Galen, true knowledge rests upon theory supported by experience; observation alone cannot rule out chance. To oversimplify, he argued that digested food is converted into blood in the liver. The blood then partakes of a life-giving principle that enters the body through the respiratory system. In giving life and nutrition to the body the blood itself is consumed.

Despite the basic errors in the classical inheritance that medieval universities perpetuated, the writings of Hippocrates and Galen did contain valuable lessons for future physicians. Hippocrates believed that

---

trans. and ed. Evan H. Hare (London, 1891). I have also used these works for identifying medical figures throughout the text, except where noted.

2. The 1254 *Ordenanzas* used the word "física," but in *Las Siete Partidas* (Parte II, Tit. ix, Ley 10) the definition of "física" is one who "preserves life and health." A papal bull of 1313, in its list of Salamancan courses, substituted the word "medicina." This is discussed in R. P. Beltran de Heredia, *Los orígenes de la Universidad de Salamanca* (Salamanca, 1953), pp. 44 ff.

3. *Ibid*., p. 43; Vicente de La Fuente, *Historia de las universidades, colegios, y demás establecimientos de enseñanza en España* (4 vols.; Madrid, 1884–1889), I, 214–221.

4. On Hippocrates, see Henry E. Sigerist, *A History of Medicine* (New York, 1961) II, 260–297. There is considerable debate over the composition and authorship of the corpus of Hippocratic works. On Galen, see Owsei Temkin, *Galenism, Rise and Decline of a Medical Philosophy* (Ithaca, N.Y., 1973).

the physician must rely on his own experience, not theory, and must consider each case separately. One learns about diseases by studying their course in specific cases; only then can general principles be deduced. Much of the huge corpus of Hippocratic works, particularly the multi-volume *Epidemics*, contained excellent detailed clinical descriptions. In Spanish medical faculties, however, two shorter works formed the basis of the curriculum: the *Prognostics*, a careful study of clinical procedures, disease symptoms and their classifications, and the means to evaluate them; and the *Aphorisms*, a virtual synthesis of all Hippocratic wisdom from broad philosophical precepts to concrete practical advice. In all his works Hippocrates emphasized the body's ability to heal itself; his usual recommended cures consisted of diet, rest, occasionally drugs, not the bloodlettings and purges that eighteenth-century medics prescribed with such abandon. The works of Galen, though more doctrinaire, contained detailed anatomical descriptions. Although some of his assertions later proved to be erroneous, his approach nevertheless underlined the need for careful observation. Thus, the weakness of relying on Hippocrates and Galen for the basis of a medical education lay less in their content than in the exclusion of practical experience and new material that might have supplemented the knowledge gleaned from the texts. Hippocrates himself no doubt would have deplored the manner in which his texts were used.

The reluctance to replace Hippocrates and Galen until late in the eighteenth century was based less on the merit of the texts themselves than on the fact that these two authors represented the authority of the ancients. During the Middle Ages Galenic medicine was accepted as the basis of medical knowledge, as the correct system, even if some of his specific assertions were incorrect. The Renaissance preoccupation with returning to the original Greek and Latin sources only increased its status. Since much early opposition to Galenic medicine came from Protestants on religious grounds, its position in the universities of Catholic Spain became even more secure. By the eighteenth century Galenic medicine was closely associated with Aristotelian metaphysics. As a result, the question of accuracy in Hippocrates and Galen was eclipsed by the more basic issue of whether universities would support a traditional world view.[5]

5. Temkin, *Galenism*, esp. pp. 167–168; Lester S. King, "Medical Theory and Practice at the Beginning of the 18th Century," *Bulletin of the History of Medicine*, XLVI (1972), 1.

For a time, to be sure, medicine in Spain had been anxious to incorporate the latest scientific progress. The sixteenth century, the *siglo de oro*, was the apogee of academic medicine in Spain. Public dissections, which had been held occasionally since the thirteenth century, became more common. The medical faculties at Salamanca and Valladolid ranked among the best in Europe. Newly created universities such as Alcalá de Henares, a project of Cardinal Ximenes de Cisneros, included well-endowed medical faculties. A chair of anatomy was established at Salamanca in 1561. According to the university statutes, this professor was to perform six dissections a year and to use Vesalius (1514–1564) as his guide.[6]

The ready acceptance of Vesalius only eighteen years after the publication of his *De humani corporis fabrica* was indicative of the modern spirit that permeated Spanish education in the sixteenth century, for Vesalius was the first to challenge directly the authority of Galen.[7] He not only pointed out specific errors in Galen, but also challenged his basic methodology of dissecting animal instead of human cadavers. Although Vesalius threatened little in contemporary medical practice, his work did demonstrate the value of observation over authority. Elsewhere in Spain, Michael Servetus (1511–1553), a clergyman, provided a little-noticed description of pulmonary circulation in a theological tract. Thus, during the sixteenth-century academic medicine cast aside tradition and opened itself to the empirical approach of modern science.

Numerous hospitals were also founded in the sixteenth and seventeenth centuries. For years convents and monasteries had been caring for the sick, but Philip II established royal hospitals to offer more professional care. In 1587 he built the Hospital General in Madrid, using the combined resources of several less efficient religious establishments. That same year the Hospital de la Pasión, a women's hospital founded in 1465, was legally attached to the Hospital General. When new quarters were constructed in 1647 a narrow alley separated the men's and women's wards. In the years to come such royal hospitals would prove to be extremely important in providing an alternative for training future doctors as well as to care for patients. Hospitals also offered their practitioners a sure source of income, valuable and

6. George M. Addy, *The Enlightenment in the University of Salamanca* (Durham, N.C., 1966), p. 44. Vesalius was the Crown physician at the time.

7. On Vesalius, see C. D. O'Malley, *Andreas Vesalius of Brussels, 1514–1564* (Berkeley, 1965); Lester S. King, *The Growth of Medical Thought* (Chicago, 1963), pp. 139 ff.; Temkin, *Galenism*, pp. 138–141.

varied experience, and the opportunity to experiment with new medications and techniques.[8]

Toward the middle of the seventeenth century, however, Spanish medicine began its decline. As early as 1625 Galen once again became the basic anatomy text at Salamanca.[9] The number of students studying medicine in universities dropped substantially; in 1785, only 706 of the more than ten thousand students in Spanish universities were studying medicine.[10] No further changes took place in degree requirements or textbooks until the 1770s. Public dissections became less and less frequent. According to an eighteenth-century professor of anatomy, many Salamancan professors "feared" that subject. Moreover, it was all but impossible to obtain a sufficient number of cadavers, and students were not required to attend dissections.[11]

By the eighteenth century all accounts agree that Spanish medicine was generally backward, ineffective, even harmful. An English visitor, for example, referred to physicians as "a distemper fatal in the country."[12] University medicine continued to rely on Hippocrates, Galen, and Avicenna. Students spent long hours in the classroom classifying parts of the body, proving metaphysical explanations of phenomena in good syllogistic form, and memorizing lengthy passages in Latin. Rarely did a student come in contact with a cadaver, or even a patient. What little original thinking that did occur in medical faculties was devoted to passionate defenses of one theoretical system over another. The physician who developed a new theory of the "vital force" in man, or of the relationship between the body and the soul, was far more respected than the man who developed a new cure or method of healing a wound. Small wonder that a doctor from Cartagena complained that students left the university "fanatics to theories."[13] To

8. On royal hospitals, see Antonio Soroa y Tineda, "El Hospital General de Madrid como escuela, templo, tradición y fortaleza señera de la medicina de la villa y corte," *Gaceta médica española*, XXXVIII (1964), 337–342; Julian de la Villa, "Historia del Hospital General, hoy Provincial," *Anales de la Real Academia Nacional de Medicina*, LXVIII (1956), 51–61; José Alvarez-Sierra, *Historia de la cirugía española* (Madrid, 1961), pp. 12–14.

9. Addy, *The Enlightenment in . . . Salamanca*, p. 43.

10. La Fuente, *Historia de las universidades*, IV, 153.

11. Archivo Histórico Nacional (Madrid), Sección de Consejos Suprimidos, Legajo 5464 (hereinafter cited as AHN, Consejos, Leg. 5464), Expediente 14, Representación de Francisco Antonio de Zunzunegui, 1783.

12. Richard Cumberland to the Earl of Hillsborough, July 21, 1780, quoted in Richard B. Morris, *The Peacemakers* (New York, 1965), p. 61.

13. Archivo Histórico General de Simancas, Sección de Secretaría de Gracia y Justicia, Leg. 404 (Old Series, Leg. 990) (hereinafter cited AGS, Gracia y Justicia, Leg. 404 [990]), Manifesto de algunas reflexiones ventajosas al . . . mejor estado de la

make matters worse, medicine ranked last among the university faculties. As a result, the faculty of medicine was frequently a refuge for students unable to succeed in another discipline.

In addition to an academic degree, the law required future doctors to spend two years as an apprentice to a practicing physician. Most doctors who took in such apprentices, however, taught them little, preferring only to have the young man carry his bags and perform simple tedious chores. Rarely would the apprentice actually administer medications, much less follow one case through from beginning to end. Even so, it was not unusual for a candidate to be excused from the required two years.[14]

Although Spain's best doctors ranked with the best in Europe, medical practice as a whole was not only criticized by liberal reformers but was held in popular contempt. Writers of the time frequently pictured physicians reciting Latin phrases they did not understand in order to impress their patients. As in every age, there were complaints that physicians were more eager to secure honors and influential friends than to build a more healthy society. Many medical men built their reputations on a single remedy that they prescribed for every ailment.[15] Equally disturbing was the severe shortage of doctors. Antonio Domínguez Ortiz estimates that by the eighteenth century there were only about four thousand physicians in all of Spain.[16] The shortage affected rural areas the worst.

---

medicina, que al . . . Conde de Floridablanca . . . presenta El Doctor Martín Rodón y Bell, Feb. 7, 1777. On poor academic conditions, see also Antonio Pérez de Escobar, *Medicina Patria o Elementos de la Medicina Práctica de Madrid* (Madrid, 1788), pp. xxiv ff.; Feijóo, *Teatro crítico*, tom. I, disc. 3; tom. VII disc. 14; tom. VIII, disc. 3, in *Obras*, II, 33–55; III, 462–472; and I, 438–441, respectively; Marañón, "Las ideas biológicas," p. cv; García del Real, *Historia de la Medicina en España*, pp. 418–427.

14. AGS, Gracia y Justicia, Leg. 404 (990), Al . . . Conde de Floridablanca representa el Dr. Vicente Crespo, Médico Titular de . . . Brihuega, Dec. 30, 1784; Dictamen del fiscal, Oct. 18, 1771, in AHN, Consejos, Leg. 1035, Expediente 1, Parte 5, Consulta del Consejo de Castilla satisfaciendo a una Real Orden que expone lo que se le ofrece esta facultad, y propone los medios que se podran adoptar a este fin, Aug. 23, 1774. This four-hundred page *consulta*, hereinafter cited as Consulta sobre cirugía, traces the legal history of surgical education since the 1740s and paraphrases almost verbatim innumerable relevant documents. Since the consulta has no pagination I shall refer to the particular document summary in the report.

15. On the state of popular medicine, see AHN, Consejos, Leg. 924, Exp. 22, Parte 1, Informe de los Alcaldes mayores examinadores del . . . Protomedicato por lo correspondiente a . . . Cirugía, Oct. 31, 1782 (hereinafter cited as AHN, Consejos, Leg. 924, Informe del Protomedicato—Cirugia); AGS, Gracia y Justicia, Leg. 404 (911), Representación del Dr. Vicente Crespo, Dec. 30, 1784; Feijóo, *Teatro crítico*, tom. VIII, disc. 10, in *Obras*, IV, 83–134, and *Cartas eruditas*, tom. V, carta 21, pp. 396–424; Kany, *Life and Manners*, p. 239.

16. *La sociedad española*, p. 168.

The professional, university-trained physician discussed thus far never represented more than a small minority of the available medical practitioners. Since only the wealthy could afford to retain a professional physician, most Spaniards—indeed, most Europeans—were compelled to turn to surgeons and barbers for assistance. Thus, medical practice before the nineteenth century encompassed not only the graduates of university faculties of medicine but also a wide variety of craftsmen who had learned their trade only as apprentices.

The distinction betwen physician and surgeon had its roots in the medical classics inherited from the ancients. The Hippocratic Oath apparently prohibited cutting for stones, and Galen described surgery as "a mode of treatment," not a profession in itself.[17] Islamic medicine intensified the distinction since the Moslem physician routinely delegated surgical procedure to others. Once medicine became a part of the medieval university, the division became complete: the physician was a professional, familiar with the classics and possessing an academic degree; the surgeon, on the other hand, was an uneducated craftsman who worked with his hands.

As a result, the surgeon consistently occupied a lowly position. Lacking formal education and the butt of frequent jokes, the surgeon was as despised by the physician as he was feared by the public. His world of bleedings, amputations, and bone-setting seemed far removed from that of the dignified, well-dressed physician, learned in Latin and philosophy. The surgeon's visits were dreaded events, accompanied as they were by shrieks of pain, and often death. Thus, the general disdain for using one's hands combined with the sordid nature of surgery to place the surgeon in an unenviable position.

Nevertheless, although he lacked a formal education, the surgeon often had greater practical experience than the university physician. Having acquired his skill first as an apprentice, then as a practitioner, he was often less wedded to theories and outdated principles than the man who had learned his trade in the classroom. In an age when practical medicine consisted largely of prescribing herbs, treating wounds, and the ever-present bloodletting, little theoretical knowledge was really necessary.

17. Galen is quoted in Garrison, *An Introduction to the History of Medicine*, p. 143. Scholars have long debated the passage from Hippocrates. Should the physician avoid all cutting or just this particular operation? Others have variously asserted that the passage was inserted much later, or that "cut" should be translated as "castrate." See W. H. S. Jones, ed., *Hippocrates* (Loeb Classical Library; Cambridge, Eng., 1962), pp. 293–294.

The distinction between physician and surgeon characterized all European medicine until the nineteenth century. Everywhere surgeons possessed little or no academic training and were considered members of a craft, not a learned profession. In the British Isles surgery did not win professional university status until after 1800, although individual academic chairs were founded earlier in the century in Scotland. At other universities, including Paris, the candidate for a medical degree had to swear that he would never engage in surgery.[18] French surgeons found themselves stigmatized as barbers until the 1740s when a university degree became a prerequisite to practicing surgery. Only the celebrated University of Montpellier dared to break with tradition by initiating a combined program for physician-surgeons. Thus, efforts to improve surgical practice had to include the transformation of surgery from a despised craft into a respected profession.

One of the first real efforts in Europe to improve the practice of surgery and make it a respectable profession occurred in sixteenth-century Spain. In 1561 a chair of surgery was established at the University of Salamanca. Some thirty years later a similar chair was endowed at Alcalá de Henares. Finally, in 1617, a royal decree required all university medical faculties to have chairs of surgery and anatomy. Only university-trained surgeons, or Latin surgeons, as they were called, were eligible for posts in universities, many hospitals, and with the royal family. As a result, surgery was never as separate from medicine in Spain as elsewhere, although the disputes between physicians and surgeons, and among surgeons themselves, were certainly as bitter.[19]

The royal hospitals that first appeared in the sixteenth century contributed significantly to raising the level of surgical practice. Most hospitals required surgeons on their staff to supervise the training of future practitioners. The Hospital of Antón Martín, which was estab-

18. On British surgery, see H. P. Tait, "Medical Education at the Scottish Universities to the Close of the Eighteenth Century"; and R. S. Roberts, "Medical Education and the Medical Corporations," in British Congress on the History of Medicine, *The Evolution of Medical Education in Britain*, ed. F. N. L. Poynter (London, 1966), pp. 53–68 and 69–88, respectively; Zachary Cope, *The Royal College of Surgeons of England* (Springfield, Ill., 1959); A. Logan Turner, *Story of a Great Hospital: The Royal Infirmary of Edinburgh, 1726–1929* (Edinburgh, 1937), esp. pp. 131 ff. On France, see the articles by Toby Gelfand, esp. "From Guild to Profession: The Surgeons of France in the 18th Century," *Texas Reports on Biology and Medicine*, XXXII (1974), 121–134.

19. Addy, *The Enlightenment in . . . Salamanca*, p. 44; Luis Alonso Muñoyerro, *La Facultad de Medicina en la Universidad de Alcalá de Henares* (Madrid, 1945), p. 31.

lished for patients suffering from venereal diseases, was important since that ailment was in the domain of surgery. There surgeons, not physicians, were in command.

The establishment of surgical training in universities and hospitals had a negligible effect on the profession as a whole, however. Hospital positions were few in number and difficult to obtain. In addition, most university students naturally opted for a career in medicine, with its greater social and financial benefits. As a result, many positions reserved exclusively for Latin surgeons were frequently vacant. The chair of surgery at Alcalá, for example, was unoccupied for so long that in 1725 the Crown permitted any medical graduate to apply.[20]

Thus, by the beginning of the eighteenth century, despite nominal recognition of surgery as an academic career, the vast majority of practicing surgeons still had learned their craft as apprentices. These romance surgeons, as they were known, had little formal education. Some were even illiterate. Most lacked even the most elementary understanding of human anatomy. Usually the years of apprenticeship taught little more than a few basic techniques. Small wonder that the surgeon was commonly believed to be an indigent, lazy individual who had chosen to practice surgery because he knew nothing about anything else.[21] His financial rewards were proportional to his social standing: the typical charge for a home visit was one real, less than the cost of a loaf of bread.[22]

In order to better understand the structure of Spanish medicine and the problems involved in its reform, it is necessary to examine the regulation and licensing of the profession. For Spanish medicine was governed not by universities, guilds, or governmental bodies, but rather by the Royal Protomedicato. If the requirements for practicing medicine and surgery in Spain resembled those in force throughout Europe, the legal structure of the Protomedicato was surely unique.[23]

20. AHN, Sección de Universidades y Colegios (hereinafter AHN, Universidades), Leg. 42, Carta orden, July 25, 1725. All *expedientes* of *oposiciones* in the *legajo* concerning the chair of surgery specify Latin surgeon.

21. AHN, Consejos, Leg. 924, Informe del Protomedicato—Cirugía, Oct. 31, 1782; Informe del Colegio de Cirugía de Madrid, 1753, in Consulta sobre cirugía.

22. Joseph Townsend, *A Journey Through Spain in the Years 1786 and 1787* (3 vols.; London, 1791), III, 397, cited in Georges Desdevises du Dezert, "La Richesse et la Civilisation Espagnoles au XVIIIe Siècle," *Revue Hispanique*, LXXIII (1928), 336. Price comparisons, taken from Earl J. Hamilton, *War and Prices in Spain, 1651–1800* (Cambridge, Mass., 1947), pp. 155 ff., are based on Madrid in the 1780s.

23. For a history of the Protomedicato, see Pascual Iborra, "Memoria sobre la institución del Real Proto-Medicato," *Anales de la Real Academia de Medicina*, VI (1885–1886), 183–307, 387–397, 531–532, 570–592.

The Protomedicato, probably founded in the fifteenth century, licensed all medical practitioners, arbitrated disputes between them, and punished malpractice and quackery. Its purpose was to guarantee uniformly high standards of medical practice, safeguard the public from incompetents, and protect the privileges of the practitioners themselves. The members of this board and its local delegates, all medical men themselves, were appointed by the Crown. Thus, in Spain the regulation of practitioners was traditionally separate from the school or guild that trained them. Indeed, no examiner could participate in licensing a former student.[24]

The principal activity of the Protomedicato was to license all physicians, surgeons, barbers, and pharmacists, and to define the requirements and privileges of each.[25] Throughout its history the board devoted great effort to setting distinctions among the various categories and guaranteeing that no practitioner performed any procedure for which he was not licensed. No one could practice any variety of medicine in Spain without the approval of the Protomedicato, although the frequent repetition of this dictum by the Crown suggests that it was difficult to enforce. Local examiners enforced the standards set by the board itself. The Crown made repeated efforts to discourage them from granting exceptions to all the requirements.[26] No doubt many local officials felt an unqualified practitioner was better than none at all.

In order to apply for any license from the Protomedicato, a candidate first had to certify his *limpieza de sangre* and thus legally prove that he and his ancestors had never been tainted by non-Christian blood or had been called before the Inquisition. A law of 1737 underlined the importance of this requirement by asserting that the Council of Castile would consider appeals from the Protomedicato on this ques-

24. Archivo del Real Palacio, Madrid, (hereinafter cited as ARP), Sección Administriva, Leg. 691, *Ordenanzas . . . para la ensenanza de Medicina Práctica en las Cátedras nuevemente establecidas en el Hospital General de Madrid con la denominación de Estudio Real de Medicina Práctica* (Madrid, 1795), cap. III, art. 3. These ordinances, hereinafter cited as *Ordenanzas para el Estudio de Medicina Práctica* (1795), contain much on the traditional structure of the Protomedicato. On its founding, see also Iborra, "Memoria," pp. 186–190.

In Spanish America, on the other hand, the Protomedicato was less separate from academic medicine. Indeed, the senior professor of medicine was customarily the first protomédico. (See John Tate Lanning, "Legitimacy and *Limpieza de Sangre* in the Practice of Medicine in the Spanish Empire," *Jahrbuch für Geschichte von Staat, Wirtschaft und Gesellschaft Lateinamerikas*, IV [1967], 40.)

25. *Nov. Rec.*, VIII, x, 1.

26. *Ibid.*, VIII, x, 2, 5, and 7.

tion alone.[27] Despite the restrictions, however, many such "tainted" individuals apparently practiced medicine unmolested.

The most prestigious medical profession was that of *médico*, or physician. He needed a bachelor of arts degree, four years of medicine in a university, and two years of practice with a licensed physician during which he could not practice medicine by himself.[28] By requiring a period of apprenticeship, the Protomedicato implied that theoretical knowledge, as certified by an academic degree, was not enough. The examination itself consisted of oral questions based on Hippocrates, Galen, and Avicenna, and a practical session in a hospital in which the candidate had to discuss particular patients. No conditional or restricted licenses were permitted. In theory, the system should have licensed only educated, competent physicians. However, later laws suggest that local boards all too often excused the candidate from the two years of practice.

The candidate for surgeon needed only to have practiced four years beside an approved surgeon. He was to have some knowledge of Hippocrates, Galen, and the medieval surgeon Guy de Chauliac (1300–1367), but, unlike the candidate for physician, he was not expected to have memorized his studies. (In practice, the Protomedicato usually passed a candidate if he could recite a few lines of Hippocrates or Galen.) After chairs of surgery were established in universities, two years of academic work could replace two of the years of practice. In 1603 the total period of training was increased to five years. Barbers had only to pass an examination; midwives were not examined at all until 1750. During the eighteenth century a wide variety of new titles were introduced—bleeder, dentist, occulist—each with its own examination and fees.[29] Nevertheless, it was to the credit of the Protomedicato that it realized the value of practical experience more than the universities did.

The variety in the requirements led to clearer distinctions between the types of medical men. These distinctions were not insignificant, for they determined salaries, the type of job open to the individual, and would, in the eighteenth century, become an important factor in medical reform. Physicians were limited to internal diseases such as fevers. Surgeons could only cure external problems such as wounds,

27. *Ibid.*, VIII, x, 9. See also Lanning, "Legitimacy."

28. Requirements are contained in *Nov. Rec.*, VIII, x, 4, 6, and 7.

29. *Ibid.*, VIII, x, 9; AHN, Consejos, Leg. 924, Informe del Protomedicato—Cirugía, Oct. 31, 1792; Informe del Colegio de Cirugía de Madrid, 1753, in Consulta sobre cirugía.

skin problems, venereal disease, and fractures. Barbers could pull teeth, bleed, and scarify. It is worth noting that although only Latin surgeons were eligible for certain prestigious positions, anyone licensed as a surgeon could practice all aspects of that art. There were severe penalties for anyone who exceeded his authority.[30] Unfortunately, there were many patients with a variety of symptoms (*afectos mixtos*) whose problem could not easily be defined as internal or external. As a result, much of the litigation before the Protomedicato concerned physicians who had allegedly practiced surgery and vice versa.[31]

The Protomedicato jealously guarded its jurisdiction over all medical matters from attacks by universities and local guilds, and from the tendency of the Council of Castile to overrule it. For one thing, it derived most of its income from licensing fees. In addition, the board felt itself best qualified to judge the unnecessarily complex cases that came before it. Should a candidate with the required medical courses still have to take an arts degree? Could the years of practice precede the years of university studies? Although only a small number of cases were examined, it would appear that the Protomedicato tended to observe the letter of the law more closely than did the Council of Castile.[32]

In addition to licensing individuals, the Royal Protomedicato was responsible for safeguarding the public from quacks, ineffective or dangerous medications, and misleading advertising. Documents of specific cases suggest that the creator of a new drug had to obtain permission of the Protomedicato before advertising it. Statements by doctors testifying to the drug's effectiveness usually accompanied the petition.[33] Sometimes doctors refused to reveal the contents of new drugs to preserve their monopoly. To remedy this, the Crown provided that the sample would be sealed until ten years after the death of the inventor.[34] From time to time officials also sought the advice of the Protomedicato in regard to specific local problems. On one oc-

30. *Nov. Rec.*, VIII, x, 3, 5, 6, and 8.

31. AGS, Gracia y Justicia, Leg. 405 (991), Real cédula, Nov. 21, 1737. Also, AHN, Consejos, Leg. 1845, contains many such cases that were appealed from the Protomedicato to the Council of Castile—in spite of the decree against such appeals.

32. ARP, Leg. 689, Exposición del Protomedicato, Oct. 12, 1704; AGS, Secretaría de Hacienda, Leg. 953, Expediente sobre Eusevio Xavier de Castro, May 19, 1775, and Representación de Manuel de la Raya sobre usurpaciones de la jurisdición y atribuciones del Real Protomedicato, 1774. The latter document, written by the president of the Protomedicato of Castile, enumerates many so-called abuses by higher authorities.

33. AGS, Gracia y Justicia, Leg. 404 (989), Expediente de Luisa Rosada, 1771, et al.

34. AHN, Consejos, Leg. 812, Exp. 2, Real cédula, May 20, 1788.

casion the board recommended that the Crown provide fresh vegetables to the poor to help combat a type of fever (*las tercinas*, or tertian ague). In this case pamphlets were circulated to local doctors.[35] Other actions to benefit the public were more mundane. In 1770 the Protomedicato ordered a group of barbers to change the signs outside their shops so the public would not confuse them with surgeons.[36] Thus, given the wide jurisdiction of the Protomedicato, it is not surprising that the College of San Carlos would meet with opposition when it began to assume many of the board's functions.

In addition to the universities and the Protomedicato, whose role in regulating medicine is clear, there were also innumerable guilds (*gremios*), colleges (*colegios*), and brotherhoods (*confradías*) that governed local medicine.[37] Unfortunately, documents in official archives contain only occasional references to such institutions, so knowledge of them remains somewhat vague. At any rate, in many localities one had to be a member of the respective college or brotherhood before he could practice his respective branch of medicine. The college not only monopolized the profession but also offered its members aid in times of personal hardship, provided opportunities for collective acts of piety, often furnished instruction in the craft for new members, and served as a fraternal organization. Needless to say, the brotherhoods had frequent jurisdictional disputes with the Protomedicato over which body had the final voice as to who could practice medicine. The privileges of a brotherhood ultimately depended upon the charter it had received from the Crown. The most insignificant departure from the charter required royal approval.[38]

The most significant brotherhood was the guild of surgeons and bloodletters (*sangradores*), the Confradía of San Cosme y San Damian, named after two doctors martyred under Diocletian. Chartered in 1583, the Confradía monopolized all surgical practice in Madrid; membership in the Confradía was a prerequisite to practicing surgery in

35. AHN, Consejos, Leg. 11934, Exp. 4, Informe del Protomedicato . . . para endagar las causas y método curativo de las tercianas, 1785; *Memorial Literario Instructivo y Curioso de la Corte de Madrid*, Aug. 1786, pp. 514 ff. The *Médicos de cámara* (king's physicians, an honorary title in many cases) were also consulted; they recommended quinine.

36. AHN, Consejos, Leg. 783, Exp. 1, Dictamen del Protomedicato, March 18, 1779.

37. The three terms are used interchangeably; *colegio* in this sense does not refer to a school. The best short description is in La Fuente, *Historia de la universidades*, IV, 237.

38. AGS, Secretaría de Hacienda, Leg. 952, Expediente sobre la Confradía de San Cosme y San Damian, Dec. 9, 1772. In this case the Confradía sought to transfer funds from a fiesta to benefit widows.

that city. Most, if not all, of its members were romance surgeons (no university education) and bleeders. During the eighteenth century the organization became very conservative as it saw its privileges threatened by new institutions. The brotherhood offered no formal training to its members, and it opposed the establishment of any schools that would not be subject to it. Campomanes accused it of being far more interested in its own members than in the health of the people of Madrid.[39]

Similar brotherhoods, usually of surgeons, monopolized medical practice in other cities and towns with frequently the same effect. In the Aragonese city of Teruel, one college, founded by Philip IV, regulated medicine, surgery, and pharmacy, in an uncommon unification of the branches of medicine. In 1775 numerous citizens begged the Crown to annul the college's charter, claiming that it had prevented any new methods from being introduced. One man complained he had had a fever for six months but no one even visited him.[40]

Such complaints were common during the eighteenth century throughout Europe, for medical training simply failed to keep pace with the rapid growth of medical knowledge. Indeed, the more prestigious the university, the more it seemed to resist change. With few exceptions, medical faculties everywhere, including those at Paris, Oxford, and Cambridge, still relied on Hippocrates and Galen. Systematic clinical experience was virtually nonexistent; specialization was unknown.

The principal exception to this dismal picture of university medicine was the University of Leyden, which came to serve as a model for reform elsewhere. Under the direction of Hermann Boerhaave, the medical faculty there revolutionized medical education. Although some clinical training had existed since 1637, Boerhaave made the clinic the basis for the curriculum. For the first time the patient himself became the principal tool of medical pedagogy. Boerhaave taught his students to judge each case individually and to follow carefully all changes in the patient's condition as medications were applied. He

39. Dictamen de Campomanes, Oct. 19, 1771, in Consulta sobre cirugía. The consulta contains numerous other references to the Confradía. See also AHN, Consejos (Sala de Gobierno), Leg. 721, Exp. 27, La Hermandad de San Cosme y San Damian de Cirujanos y Sangradores . . . , 1777; AHN, Consejos, Leg. 1359e (Libro de Gobierno de la Sala de Alcaldes de Casa y Corte, hereinafter cited as Libro de Gobierno), Fol. 171–176, Orden, April 12, 1771; Alfredo Lapuente Mateos, "Para la historia de la hermandad de San Cosme y San Damian," *Medicamenta*, IX (1948), 97.

40. AGS, Gracia y Justicia, Leg. 404 (989), Representación del Obisbo de Teruel, Nov. 28, 1775.

believed that the true scientist bases his findings on experience, and reasons to his conclusions from what he observes, not from first principles. Under Boerhaave, students observed first-hand what their predecessors had read only in books. Students of Boerhaave, coming from all over Europe, returned home to establish similar schools: Gerard Van Swieten reorganized the Vienna medical faculty, Albrecht von Haller (1708–1777) founded a new school at the University of Goettingen in Germany, Alexander Munro established a medical faculty at the University of Edinburgh.

Boerhaave's influence spread still further through his textbooks. He believed that the ideal medical education began with the natural sciences, proceeded to anatomy, and concluded with a study of the diseased body. His major work, *Institutiones medicae*, was a careful synthesis of anatomy, physiology, and chemistry. First introduced at Leyden in 1701, it would come to replace the classical authors throughout Europe. His other major work, *Aphorisms*, a collection of practical clinical advice, became similarly popular. In addition, Gerard Van Swieten, his student, wrote five volumes of widely used commentaries on the *Aphorisms*, apparently gleaned from the master's lectures.[41]

Innovation elsewhere, however, occurred outside the universities. Hospitals and private academies sponsored public lectures and anatomical demonstrations that quickly became popular pastimes as well as valuable training for practicing physicians and surgeons. Hospitals in Madrid, Paris, and London offered formal clinical training. Private individuals, especially in England, provided lessons to selected students. Thus scientific progress was intimately tied to social change within the profession.

French surgery, supported by the Crown, probably made the most substantial advances. The University of Montpellier, already a leader in medical reform, granted the first combined degree of physician-surgeon as early as 1734, although the innovative program had difficulty attracting students for decades to come.[42] In 1743 a royal decree separated surgeons from barbers and awarded surgeons professional status by requiring them to possess a university degree. Seven years later a

41. On Boerhaave, see G. A. Lindeboom, *Herman Boerhaave: The Man and His Work* (London, 1968); Lester S. King, *The Medical World of the Eighteenth Century* (Chicago, 1958), pp. 59–122; I. Snapper, *Meditations on Medicine and Medical Education* (New York, 1956), pp. 53–83.

42. Louis Dulieu, "Pierre Chirac, sa vie, ses écrits, ses idées," *Montpellier Medical*, 3rd ser., LI (1957), 767–786.

French surgical college, which had sponsored lectures for several decades, acquired regular academic status. Attendance there became mandatory in order to practice surgery in Paris. In 1774 the college established its own clinic modeled on that at Leyden.[43]

Elsewhere, surgeons were less successful in acquiring full professional status, although they made considerable progress. English surgeons became completely separate from barbers in 1745. The progressive University of Edinburgh initiated clinical instruction in surgery in 1768.[44]

The new surgeons were eager to apply their superior knowledge by attempting new procedures. In the past the surgeon had dealt only with external, "visible" problems, such as wounds, abscesses, venereal disease, and skin diseases; his procedures had been limited to bloodletting, purges, bone-setting, and amputations. During the eighteenth century, however, surgery began to realize its potential for alleviating internal maladies. As a result, the new surgeons attempted daring operations in which they cut into the body to remove all manner of stones and tumors. Thus, the gradual professionalization of surgery led to a substantial redefinition of its function.

To be sure, internal surgery could not become the common remedial science it is today until well into the nineteenth century. Without a safe, effective anesthesia, speed was essential, often at the expense of thoroughness. Since the necessity for antiseptic conditions was unknown, postoperative infection was common. Often subjects of successful operations fell victim to shock or hemorrhaging. Thus, the advanced procedures of innovative surgeons were of limited practical value: technique had surpassed science. Yet were it not for the minority of surgeons who saw themselves as scientists and who demonstrated the full potential of their art, the dramatic advances of later centuries might never have occurred.[45]

Yet, in Spain, as elsewhere in eighteenth-century Europe, both medicine and surgery presented a striking contrast. On the one hand was a small number of innovative scientists familiar with the latest medical developments. On the other was the large majority of prac-

43. Toby Gelfand, "Empiricism and Eighteenth-Century Surgery," *Bulletin of the History of Medicine*, XLIV (1973), 40–53, and "The Hospice of the Paris College of Surgery (1774–1793), 'A Unique and Valuable Institution,'" *Bulletin of the History of Medicine*, XLVII (1973), 375–393.

44. For England and Scotland, see n. 18, above.

45. See Frederick F. Cartwright, *The Development of Modern Surgery* (New York, 1967), esp. pp. 12–14.

titioners, poorly trained, ignorant of recent discoveries, often incompetent. Spain was no exception. According to the medical historian Antonio Hernández Morejón, Spanish surgeons successfully performed such advanced operations as repairing hernias, cutting tissue covering the cornea of the eye (pterigium), removing cataracts, tying off arteries, removing stones, and removing cancerous parts of the eye and tongue.[46] Yet, for the most part, bleeding and purgation remained the universal cures, and much debate revolved around the best methods of administering them. Patients expected the traditional remedies, and doctors were eager to oblige.

In rural areas medicine was almost barbaric. Most villages had one practitioner at most and could not afford to investigate his certification too carefully. Some practitioners, no doubt, were very dedicated. One such man, who had only a physician's license, was brought before the Protomedicato for opening an abscess with a lancet, though a surgeon was miles away.[47] Yet the board's vigilance was warranted, for quacks and charlatans–plus incompetent licensed practitioners–were everywhere. Tourniquets were left on amputated stumps for days. Bloodletters frequently bled their patients to death. A midwife castrated the male infants she delivered. Small wonder, then, that the medical arts were the object of scorn.[48]

Spanish hospitals, though atrocious by contemporary standards, were probably no worse than hospitals elsewhere. Indeed, at a time when one went to a hospital only if he were near death, or had no one to care for him, the mortality rate was surprisingly low.[49] The position of chief physician or chief surgeon in a major hospital such as the Madrid Hospital General was well paid and quite prestigious. A patient, particularly one with an "interesting" ailment, probably received better care there than he would have had at home. Indeed, by the end of the century most medical research was carried on in royal hospitals. On the other hand, the majority of hospital patients, particularly the very poor, were crowded, several to a bed, into small

46. Antonio Hernández Morejón, *Historia bibliográfica de la medicina española* (7 vols.; Madrid, 1842–1852), VI, 284.

47. AHN, Consejos, Leg. 1845, Exp. 10, Expediente sobre Fernando Yebra, 1797.

48. AHN, Consejos, Colección de Reales Cédulas, No. 606, Orden del Consejo, Jan. 24, 1783; Sociedad Vascongada de los Amigos del País, *Colección de Extractos de las Juntas Generales* (1789–1791), quoted in Barriola, *Las Amigos del País*, pp. 117–28; Sarrailh, *La España ilustrada*, p. 107, citing José Celestino Mutis.

49. According to the *Guía de forasteros* (Madrid, 1804), cited in Desdevises du Dezert, "Les institutions," pp. 359–360, of some 35,594 patients who entered the three principal Madrid hospitals during 1803, 27,990 left cured, 4,135 died, and 2,469 remained at the end of the period.

rooms where the lack of food and fresh air was more harmful than the illness that put them there. In 1792 the Crown even found it necessary to forbid hospitals to accept contributions of clothing from the relatives of persons who had just died of contagious diseases.[50]

Unfortunately, the very bodies entrusted with regulating medicine often contributed to the low level of everyday practice by their excessive preoccupation with the security and privileges of their members. The Protomedicato itself seemed less concerned with defending the public against bad medicine than it was with protecting physicians from those who would reform it or deflect its fees and privileges.

The *protomédicos*, physicians all, were particularly determined to keep surgery and pharmacy in a subordinate position. In 1764 the board prohibited all surgeons, even Latin surgeons, from administering bleedings and purgations, the two most common treatments, except in the presence of physicians. When called upon to explain its decree, the Protomedicato stated its attitude toward surgeons all too clearly. Only the physician, it declared, could prescribe cures because his background of Latin and philosophy enabled him to fully comprehend the laws of nature that governed diseases. The surgeon, on the other hand, was only useful when the case called for "application of hands"—but under a physician's direction. Four years later the Protomedicato scornfully dismissed a proposal to teach surgeons anatomy. Not only did the surgeon have no need for such "theory," but the course would probably be too difficult for most surgeons to comprehend.[51]

Yet there was cause for optimism. Spain's best doctors ranked with the best in Europe; even Spanish medicine as a whole may well have been less behind the rest of Europe than concerned Spaniards believed it to be. During the last quarter of the seventeenth century a new breed of university physicians known as *novatores* had begun to challenge Galen and criticize the backward state of Spanish medicine. By 1700 there was public debate on the state of the art. Even less vocal critics were not unaware of modern thought. In a manner typical of the eclectic nature of Spanish academe, many professors had synthesized Harvey's doctrine of the circulation of the blood with the medical theories of Galen, thereby accepting new knowledge without

50. AHN, Consejos, Colección de Reales Cédulas, No. 1036, Real Bando, Dec. 4, 1792. On poor hopsital conditions in general, see AGS, Gracia y Justicia, Leg. 404 (990), Reflexiones del Dr. Martín Rodón y Bell, Feb. 7, 1777; Pérez de Escobar, *Medicinia Patria*, pp. 42–43.

51. Informe del Protomedicato, 1768, in Consulta sobre cirugía.

discarding the traditional Galenic system. At the University of Valencia anatomical dissections continued on a regular basis.[52]

After 1700 even a cursory glance at Spanish critics reveals that many Spaniards, both professional and lay, were keenly aware of the decadence into which medicine had fallen. Father Feijóo and Martín Martínez were probably the most influential in publicizing the abuses and the widespread ignorance, but they were not alone. During the second half of the century many doctors and laymen in all parts of Spain wrote unsolicited appeals to the Protomedicato and the Council of Castile.[53] These "average citizens" described the abuses and begged for some kind of reform. Their suggestions—prizes for saving the most lives, avoiding arguments in the classroom, government regulations against air pollution—varied from the very farsighted to the vastly impractical. But the widely felt need for change that such appeals exhibited is convincing evidence that the reformist spirit was not limited to a few ilustrados in Madrid.

The reformist spirit, the productive research, the popular interest, and the educational innovation that represented the best of eighteenth-century medicine took place outside, and often in spite of, the universities. Such progressive physicians as Martín Martínez and Andrés Piquer (discussed in the previous chapter) made their impact upon government officials and private doctors more than upon university professors. The Economic Societies, for example, published many papers on medical topics, from infant care to proper nutrition. The Basque Society noted that medicine and surgery were among the most important fields it should encourage.[54] The medical sciences were also a popular topic in the maturing popular press. In addition to the specialized *Efemérides Barométrico-médicas Matritenses*, the *Memorial Literario Instructivo y Curioso de la Corte de Madrid* devoted a monthly section to "Surgical Observations." These usually consisted of specific case studies. Meanwhile, the Crown took steps to improve public health standards. By the end of the century the physicians of the royal family regularly visited assigned districts of Madrid.[55]

Most critics agreed that the principal shortcomings of Spanish medicine were the lack of emphasis on observation as opposed to

52. López Pinero, "Harvey's Doctrine."

53. On Feijóo and Martín Martínez, see Chap. I. The *representaciones* and *informes* cited in describing the state of medicine are examples of these appeals.

54. Barriola, *Los Amigos del País*, pp. 49, 60–82, quotes extensively from Society records.

55. ARP, Leg. 689, Disposiciones generales—Planes, 1800–1805.

theory and the almost total ignorance of human anatomy. As a result, one of the best indications of a progressive outlook came to be frequent dissections of human cadavers. To be sure, better knowledge of human anatomy was not a panacea for eighteenth-century surgery, given the limitations discussed earlier. But since anatomy symbolized observation over theory and the arrival of surgery as a profession, not a craft, its role in medical reform was of utmost importance.

Philip V endowed the first non-university chair of anatomy in 1701 at the Hospital General of Madrid. The lectures and demonstrations were open to the public. Four years later the Crown established a theater for such demonstrations at the urging of Martín Martínez. Later in the century the instruction became more formal. The fact that highly reputed anatomists such as Martín Martínez himself were appointed to the position did much to increase the prestige of that science. Many students who studied at the Hospital General went on to important posts in the military, education, and the royal household.[56] So great a success was the instruction that Ferdinand VI appointed assistants for the instructor. Other hospitals in Madrid and elsewhere later created their own chairs of anatomy.

Indeed, there seems to have been agreement on the part of both medical reformers and government officials that one could not look to the universities for innovation and progress. Numerous new institutions came into existence to teach, to do research, and to regulate the profession itself. One could attribute this anti-university feeling to envy when uttered by uneducated surgeons, but the most outspoken critics of university medicine were themselves graduates of Spanish faculties of medicine. Martín Martínez, for example, studied at Alcalá; Andrés Piquer at Valencia.

Among the private efforts to complement the universities were the academies of medicine. The Society of Medicine of Seville, which became a model for later groups, was founded in 1696. Though started by a group of doctors who felt themselves snubbed socially by the university physicians, it quickly acquired a reputation for scholarship and research. The society presented public lectures on modern writers

56. The chair of anatomy was held by José Arboleda, Pedro Martín Martínez, Bernardo López Araujo, Juan Gámez, and Pedro Custodio Gutiérrez. Gámez had studied abroad at royal expense; Custodio Gutiérrez was later president of San Carlos. A remarkable number of prominent physicians and surgeons studied there, including Juan Gámez, according to the biographies in Alvarez-Sierra, *Historia de la Cirugía española*. See also Luis Sánchez Granjel, *Anatomía española de la illustración* ("Cuadernos de Historia de la Medicina Española"; Salamanca, 1963), pp. 20–21.

and clinical discoveries and held frequent anatomical demonstrations. It even admitted physicians and surgeons as equals. The University of Seville accused it of contradicting Aristotle and Galen—which it no doubt did—but the Crown consistently supported the society. However, the University of Seville retained its monopoly to grant degrees.[57]

The Academy of Medicine of Madrid was formed in 1732 to promote medical progress in Spain and further the scholarship of its members. In public sessions members held demonstrations and gave lectures. The Madrid academy also held private sessions to discuss individual clinical cases submitted to it, current medical problems such as an epidemic or abortion, and to render advice to government bodies such as the Council of Castile. Membership in the academy became a coveted honor. By the end of the century most of its members had important positions in hospitals, the royal household, schools, or the Protomedicato. Its members came from all parts of Spain, and, occasionally, from the American colonies. Similar academies soon existed in other principal cities.[58]

The government also played a significant role in developing institutions that threatened the traditional powers of the universities, the Protomedicato, and the guilds. Indeed, one of the paradoxes of eighteenth-century Spain is that while reformers endeavored to increase royal authority by restricting autonomous institutions, they simultaneously created new bodies that possessed virtually the same degree of independence. Thus, it would appear that the Crown tended to judge specific institutions rather than to follow broad principles.

In 1748 Ferdinand VI created a "college" of surgery in Madrid as proposed by three prominent surgeons.[59] Like other medical academies,

57. Jovellanos, *Informe, . . . sobre medicina.*

58. "Estatutos de la Real Academia Médica de Madrid," "Noticia histórica del origen, progressos, y estado actual de la Real Academia Médica de Madrid," and "Catálogo de los individuos de la Real Academia Médica de Madrid," in *Memorias de la Real Academia Médica de Madrid*, I (1797), i–iii; AGS, Gracia y Justicia, Leg. 405 (992), Nota de los trabajos . . . en la Real Academia Médica-Práctica de Barcelona, 1787–1788.

59. The three were Tomás Duchesnay, First Surgeon of the King, Mateo Gierro, First Surgeon of the Hospital of San Juan de Dios, and Juan de Dios López, Surgeon of the Royal Family.

This account of the college and the controversies that followed is based on Consulta sobre cirugia; AGS, Secretaría de Hacienda, Leg. 549, Estatutos del Real Colegio de Profesores Cirujanos de Madrid, 1747, and Representación de Pedro Joseph Canizares en nombre del Real Colegio de Cirujanos, 1748. On the suppression of the surgical guild, see also Lapuente Mateos, "Para la historia de la Hermandad de San Cosme y San Damian." The educational aspects of the college will be discussed in the following chapter.

the college was empowered to select its own members, hold public lectures, and train students in surgery. But the college differed from other academies in that membership in the college automatically entitled a man to practice surgery. This, of course, was a direct threat to both the Protomedicato and the Confradía of San Cosme and San Damian. Moreover, it marked a significant departure from Spanish tradition whereby the right to license was always distinct from the right to grant degrees. No Spanish university possessed the power to license doctors.

Until its authority was threatened, the Royal Protomedicato had supported the efforts to improve surgery. Protomédicos sat on the college's board of examiners and had actively supported the chair of anatomy at the Hospital General.[60] The board insisted on its right to license all practicing surgeons, however, and maintained that all students approved by the college would also have to be approved by the Protomedicato. The college protested, declaring that the examinations given by the Protomedicato were ludicrous anyway, that a board of physicians knew nothing about surgery, and that, in any case, the standards of the college were higher than those of the Protomedicato. The Council of Castile decided against the college, however, in 1749. Henceforth, the college would have the same privileges as the Seville academy, that is, it could do everything but grant licenses and degrees.

The dispute with the Confradía of San Cosme and San Damian was more complex, for the very nature of surgery as a craft or an academic profession was at stake. The Confradía, as we have seen, consisted largely of romance surgeons and included among its members many barber shop owners who practiced minor surgery from time to time. The members of the college, on the other hand, were the elite of the profession. Many held royal appointments at court or in hospitals. They intended for their members to have some theoretical knowledge of anatomy, physiology, and pathology. As a result, they refused admission into the college to many members of the Confradía. The issue was clear. To the college, its efforts represented an attempt to raise the standards of surgical practice. To the Confradía, the college represented a self-appointed coterie trying to monopolize the profession.

This time the Council of Castile gave the college complete support. It thwarted an attempt by the Confradía to erect its own college and

60. Iborra, "Memoria," pp. 274–275.

suppress the existing one, and agreed that surgeons needed a good theoretical background before beginning their practice.

During the reign of Charles III the guild met its final defeat. The Conde de Campomanes, fiscal of the Council of Castile, opposed all guilds and felt there was no reason for surgeons and barbers to be united in the first place.[61] In 1764, as a result of his campaign against the medical "establishment," the Council of Castile forbade the Confradía of San Cosme and San Damian to license any surgeons. Three years later the Council restricted the once powerful guild to religious and social activities.

Even so, Campomanes did not stop his attack on institutions he believed were impeding medical progress. His convincing arguments that such a surgical college should, indeed, license its own students were valuable in winning support for San Carlos. He opposed the proliferation of medical titles; those of physician, surgeon, and pharmacist were enough. And in 1771 Campomanes told the Council that one of the major reforms needed in Spanish medicine was to reduce the power of the Protomedicato. He felt the Protomedicato was indifferent to the crying need for reform and interested only in maintaining the dominance of medicine over surgery and pharmacy.

The physicians of the Protomedicato lost this dominance in 1779. On the advice of his personal physicians, Charles III ordered the Protomedicato to divide itself into three separate boards: medicine, surgery, and pharmacy. Henceforth, representatives of each branch of medicine would judge the qualifications of their respective candidates. As might be expected, the reform gave way to a multitude of jurisdictional disputes.[62]

Another aspect of the changes that occurred in Spanish medicine during the second half of the eighteenth century was the growing importance of foreign studies and practitioners. Indeed, many Spanish writers explicitly set forth the state of medicine abroad as a model for Spain to follow. The Madrid college of surgery, for example, defended its existence on the basis of its similarity to a college of surgery in Paris. Spain may have been guilty of xenophobia in some things, but certainly not in medicine.

During the first half of the century the Crown encouraged foreign

61. Krebs Wilckens, *El pensamiento histórico*, p. 242.

62. AGS, Secretaría de Hacienda, Leg. 549, Expediente formado al Representación del Fiscal del Protomedicato, Dec. 5, 1780, contains the Real Resolución, May 26, 1779.

doctors to come to Spain. Many played major roles in the new institutions discussed above. José Cervi, founder of the Madrid Academy of Medicine, came from Parma with Philip's second wife, Isabel Farnese. Most of the public dissections held by the Seville academy were performed by Frenchmen.[63] The Crown apparently felt little hesitancy in appointing foreigners to important medical posts in Spain.

Other foreigners came to Spain to set up their own practice. Such was the case of Antonio de Antonio, a Neopolitan dentist who studied in Paris and London before coming to Spain.[64] Pierre Richard de Beauregard, who had studied at the Academy of Surgery in Paris and had come to Spain at the request of a Spanish military officer he had cured, became the personal surgeon of the Duke of Alba. Unfortunately, other foreigners who came were mere quacks.[65]

During the reign of Charles III many Spaniards received grants from the Crown to study abroad. Several of the early professors at San Carlos had learned their art at Montpellier or Paris.[66] Antonio Gimbernat and Mariano Rivas spent several years traveling from one European medical school to another at government expense before drawing up the plans for San Carlos. In 1779 one Juan Francisco Fabre, who was studying at Montpellier on his own when his funds ran short, petitioned the Crown for help, since the Crown was accustomed "to aid his subjects perfecting themselves at foreign universities."[67]

Thus, Spaniards were not only aware of the backward state of medicine and surgery but were taking positive steps to reform it. Individual research, medical academies, new schools, and changes in regulatory agencies all contributed to the dramatic advances made in both knowledge and practice. Although individual proposals differed, there was one thing on which all reformers agreed. No real improvement in Spanish medicine would occur until substantial changes were made in the education of physicians and surgeons. Indeed, Spanish backwardness was directly tied to the backwardness of her schools. For this reason, a review of the educational reforms of the eighteenth century, particularly as they affected medicine, is critical.

63. Sánchez Granjel, *Anatomía española*, pp. 14, 21.

64. AHN, Consejos, Leg. 783, Exp. 1, Representación de Antonio de Antonio, 1778

65. AHN, Consejos, Leg. 812, Exp. 2 and 3, Expedientes formados en virtud de . . . representación de Pedro Richard de Beauregard, 1789.

66. AGS, Secretaría de Hacienda, Leg. 952, contains several such grants for study abroad.

67. AGS, Gracia y Justicia, Leg. 404 (989), Representación de Juan Francisco Fabre, April 26, 1779. In this case the funds were not granted.

CHAPTER III

# THE REFORM OF SPANISH MEDICAL EDUCATION

MANY DIVERSE INSTITUTIONS trained physicians and surgeons in eighteenth-century Spain. A complete reform of medical education had to encompass the medical faculties of universities, the mandatory years of practice, the apprenticeship programs, and the informal instruction offered in hospitals. Despite the institutional diversity, however, the reform of medical education encompassed the same basic questions everywhere.

Curriculum reform was probably the most controversial issue. Traditionally, medicine was perceived as a body of doctrine to be learned, as in law or theology. Each course was based on a specific text of one of the classical authorities, Hippocrates, Galen, and Avicenna. By graduation the student had covered all the traditional works. Professors could easily shift from one academic chair to another since teaching a new course simply meant reading and explaining a different text.

During the eighteenth century, however, both the specific texts and the entire approach came under attack. Reformers demanded that modern texts replace the traditional ones. In addition, progressive scholars argued that since medical knowledge was becoming more complex, specific courses and instructors should concentrate upon one aspect of medicine. One class should cover anatomy, another pathology, and so forth, even if the chosen authors overlapped. Furthermore, reformers believed that students planning to study medicine needed a solid background in the natural sciences in addition to the Latin, logic, and philosophy that had traditionally formed the basis of the bachelor's degree.

The other major issue for the reformers was the proper balance between theoretical and practical studies. In the past, university medicine was restricted to the classroom, while the apprenticeships in one of the less prestigious branches of medicine included no theoretical learning whatsoever. The reformers believed that neither extreme was desirable. Academic students needed to perform a dissection if they were really to learn anatomy, to do laboratory work in order to understand chemistry, and to acquire clinical experience to care for the sick competently. Apprentices needed to know the reasons behind the procedures they learned. Memorization without experience and technique without understanding were equally dangerous.

In fact, however, the modernization of Spanish medical education in the eighteenth century was not a straightforward solution of these problems. Indeed, these difficulties were only tackled indirectly in the innumerable proposals and decisions of countless individuals and institutions put forth during the century. Reformers dedicated themselves to specific schools, universities, and academies, not to general questions of pedagogy and educational philosophy. To be sure, one institution sometimes imitated the innovation of another, sometimes by choice, sometimes by government decree. Yet Spain did not develop a national plan for medical education until well into the nineteenth century. Eighteenth-century reforms were the results of individual efforts.

Three distinct institutions were the scene of major innovation: the medical faculties of universities, classes in hospital clinics, and new colleges of surgery. In every case the Crown endeavored to combine educational reform with national standards and tighter government control. Thus, in education, as elsewhere, tradition was associated with autonomy, and innovation became tied to royal supervision and centralization.

The reform of the universities, of which medicine was only a part, has received the most attention from historians. During the sixteenth century higher education had represented the best of Spain's siglo del oro. Established institutions such as Salamanca incorporated the latest ideas of the Renaissance into the training of lawyers, physicians, and theologians. New universities such as Alcalá de Henares were established to promote the humanities. However, the early decades of the seventeenth century marked the beginning of a long period of decline and stagnation that was to endure until the reign of Charles III. Spanish intellectual life became cautious and defensive; universities concentrated on professional training that would guarantee graduates lucrative positions in the expanding bureaucracy. As a result, law became the dominant field of study. Students became preoccupied with earning the proper credentials and making the right personal connections.

Universities devoted their efforts to preserving their traditional privileges. Academic excellence suffered, as curricula became more and more out of touch with both the intellectual life of Europe and the wider needs of Spanish society. In 1625 the University of Salamanca restored Galen in place of Vesalius. No further academic changes occurred there until 1770. Campomanes remarked that Salamanca's very antiquity was partly responsible for its decadence since it had clung so long to traditional ways.[1] Other universities were similarly out of touch and out of date.

If only because of the significant progress in medical science during the preceding centuries, the medical curriculum was particularly outdated. Spanish universities were not unique, however; few universities anywhere in Europe adequately reflected the scientific advances of the seventeenth and eighteenth centuries. Throughout Europe university medicine was in a state of decline, having been all but replaced by academies and private instructors. A university education provided little to stimulate research or to arouse the curiosity of its students. Hippocrates, Galen, and Avicenna remained the basic texts at the University of Paris, for example, until the French Revolution.[2]

Medical training faced serious problems in addition to a hopelessly outdated curriculum. The requirements for the bachelor of arts degree, the prerequisite to medical studies, included extensive studies of Aristotle and Thomas Aquinas, but nothing in the natural sciences. The course in medicine, based, as has been seen, on specific authors, had no logical sequence. In most classrooms instructors merely read from the particular text. Meanwhile, the students spent most of their time in private academies (*academias particulares*) listening to fellow students. In smaller universities chairs of medicine actually went vacant

1. "Repuesta fiscal," in *Plan general de estudios dirigido a la Universidad de Salamanca por el Real y Supremo Consejo de Castilla, y mandado imprimir de su orden* (Salamanca, 1771), in Addy, *The Enlightenment in . . . Salamanca*, pp. 244–366 (hereinafter cited as *Plan general de Salamanca* [1771]). Richard Kagan has explored in depth the professionalization of Spanish universities in *Students and Society in Early Modern Spain* (Baltimore, 1974), and "The Universities in Castile, 1500–1810," in Lawrence Stone (ed.), *The University and Society* (Princeton, 1974), II, 355–405. See also Addy, *The Enlightenment in . . . Salamanca*, pp. 38–47; Sarrailh, *La España ilustrada*, pp. 142–144.

2. Erwin H. Ackerknecht, *Medicine at the Paris Hospital, 1794–1848* (Baltimore, 1967), p. 31; Hazard, *European Thought*, pp. 193–195; F. L. N. Poynter, "Medical Education in England since 1600," and Charles Coury, "The Teaching of Medicine in France from the Beginning of the Seventeenth Century," in C. D. O'Malley, *The History of Medical Education* (U.C.L.A. Forum in Medical Sciences, No. 12; Los Angeles, 1970), pp. 235–249 and 121–172, respectively.

for long periods. Others had only one chair in that important subject. In 1739 the medical faculty of Alcalá, itself quite unprogressive, complained it could not compete for students against the minor universities that granted degrees after only one or two years.[3]

Since most students sought a university degree in order to enter a professional career, the medical faculties also fell victim to the low esteem in which that profession was held. The more prestigious and lucrative careers of canon law and civil law, as well as theology, consistently attracted far more students than medicine. (Ironically, since faculties of medicine had always been small, they were the least affected by the enormous drop in student enrollment in the eighteenth century.) In 1750, for example, at Salamanca, 281 students matriculated in law (canon law and civil law), 19 in theology, and 57 in medicine. Forty years later the comparable figures were 304, 307, and 27—in spite of all the reforms. At the two other universities with a national constituency, Alcalá de Henares and Valladolid, the situation was even worse: together, in 1750, 328 students matriculated in laws, 142 in theology, but only 24 in medicine. Curiously, the medical faculties received a larger percentage of students at the smaller universities where a future career in the royal bureaucracy was less likely. At the small University of Osuna, for example, more than half the students in major faculties were studying medicine.[4]

The lack of trained physicians led to constant problems in filling the chairs of medicine. Low pay and excessively rigid standards made the situation worse. The Alcalá medical faculty, noting the perpetual vacancy of one of its chairs, plaintively asked how a man could fully dedicate himself to teaching while he was worrying about feeding his family.[5] The Council of Castile received frequent complaints that university posts were awarded solely on the basis of age. Frequent edicts ordered this practice stopped, but they met with limited success.[6]

If the state of university medicine was in need of reform, the state of university anatomy and surgery was disastrous. Charles V had first endowed a chair of anatomy at Salamanca in the sixteenth century, but

3. AHN, Consejos, Leg. 5459, Exp. 6, Plan de la Facultad de Medicina, Nov. 20, 1766 (hereinafter cited as Plan de Medicina, 1766); Resolución del Claustro de la Facultad de Medicina de la Universidad de Alcalá de Henares, June 25, 1739, quoted in La Fuente, *Historia de las universidades*, III, 330.

4. Statistics from Kagan, *Students and Society*, pp. 249–254.

5. AHN, Universidades, Signatura 1232 (hereinafter Sig. 1232), Plan de la Facultad de Medicina de Alcalá, Jan. 12, 1771.

6. AHN, Universidades, Leg. 42, Edicto de Real Consejo, Aug. 31, 1771; Acuerdo de Consejo Real, Sept. 16, 1772, et al.

it was frequently vacant. Indeed, until the 1770s students were not even required to attend classes in this all-important science. Few did. In addition, cadavers were rare, assistants unavailable, and the professor of anatomy received little pay from the university and less respect from his colleagues.[7] At Alcalá, too, the chair of anatomy was "always vacant." Indeed, the medical faculty there candidly confessed that the maligned romance surgeon knew more practical anatomy than the degree-holding physician.[8]

Theoretically, both Salamanca and Alcalá, among other universities, offered degrees in Latin surgery. But the chairs of surgery were poorly endowed, frequently vacant, and seldom attended. In 1750 one student matriculated in the program at Salamanca; none did so at Alcalá.[9] Rare was the university student who would elect such a despised, poorly paid career.

The earliest university reforms of the eighteenth century were clearly and logically initiated by the Crown. Soon after defeating his Hapsburg rival in 1713, Philip V suppressed all Catalan universities, including Lérida and Barcelona, as part of his efforts to reduce Catalan autonomy and punish the region for supporting his opponent. In their place he established the closely supervised University of Cervera in 1717 with the hope of "Castilianizing" the population. The new institution also gave Philip the opportunity of imposing a modern curriculum without countering entrenched opposition. He endowed its medical faculty with six chairs, including one of surgery and anatomy. The university statutes carefully outlined the nature of eighteen dissections that a dissector would perform each year—six to show major systems and twelve to illustrate specific organs. Wax pieces were bought from the celebrated school at Montpellier. The assigned text for the anatomy course was the *Compendio anatómico* by the famous German surgeon Lorenz Heister (1683–1758).[10] Other

7. Plan de Medicina, 1766; AHN, Consejos, Leg. 5464, Exp. 14, Representación de Francisco Antonio Zunzunegui, Feb. 6, 1778. Francisco Antonio Zunzunegui, who reformed and revitalized anatomical studies at Salamanca in the 1770s, claimed he had to teach himself the science because no formal instruction existed.

8. AHN, Universidades, Sig. 1232, Plan de la Facultad de Medicina de Alcalá, Jan. 12, 1771.

9. La Fuente, *Historia de las universidades*, III, 199.

10. Real cédula, Dec. 15, 1768, in *Cartulario de Reales Cédulas y Bulas Pontificias* (hereinafter cited as *Cartulario*), vol. IV of C. M. Ajo González y Sáinz de Zúñiga, *Historia de las universidades hispánicas: Orígines y desarrollo desde su aparición a nuestros días* (5 vols.; Madrid, 1957–1966); Ajo González, *Historia de las universidades*, V, 103–121; Desdevises du Dezert, "La Richesse et la Civilisation Espagnole," pp. 244–246; Sánchez Granjel, *Anatomía española*, p. 18.

universities would later adopt this same text as part of their reform, but not until the 1770s.

At the University of Valencia, which had boasted the best faculty of medicine in Spain during the seventeenth century, university reformers used that institution's temporary suppression between 1713 and 1720 to initiate substantial, if cautious, changes of their own. During the university's negotiations with the Crown over its restoration, the faculty of medicine observed the need to incorporate recent discoveries into the curriculum. The Valencia physicians asserted that modern medicine did not contradict the basic concepts of Hippocrates and Galen, but only added new information. Thus, it was not necessary to establish new academic chairs, but only to incorporate the new material into the existing classes. The revised constitutions for Valencia, issued in 1732, confirmed this moderate approach by requiring instruction in all modern discoveries as well as in traditional texts. In addition, the course in anatomy was now to include a remarkable twenty-six dissections each year.[11]

Despite the considerable reputations of Cervera and Valencia, no reforms followed elsewhere for several decades. Slowly, however, Spaniards became more aware of the need to change. During the 1760s demands for reform arose almost simultaneously in both the universities, particularly Salamanca, and the progressive Council of Castile.

The productive reign of Charles III marked the culmination of the Enlightenment spirit in Spanish higher education. Although eighteenth-century university reform was more a philosophy, an attitude, than a systematic program, concrete changes did occur. By the end of the century reformers had reduced the power of the *colegios mayores*, based curricula on logical divisions of content rather than authors, introduced modern texts, and established courses in the natural sciences and political economy. Thus, the reform of university faculties of medicine was part of a larger effort to renovate higher education. At the same time, however, the changes in medical education were

11. "Informe del Claustro de Medicina de Valencia sobre renovación de estudios [1721]," *Archivo Iberoamericano de Historia de la Medicina y Antropología Médica*, XIII (1961), 143–155; Ajo González, *Historia de las universidades*, V, 222–226; López Piñero, "Harvey's Doctrine," p. 234; Mariano Peset Reig and Joséf Luis Peset Reig, *La universidad española (siglos XVIII y XIX): Despotismo ilustrado y revolucción liberal* (Madrid, 1974), pp. 60–74, 259.

The University of Valencia was directly under municipal authorities and thus was relatively independent from the Crown and the Church. In addition, professors holding senior chairs had less influence than they did elsewhere.

probably the most substantial and the most necessary, for to accept the new knowledge in medicine was to reject not only specific facts but an entire philosophic tradition that rested on time-honored authorities.

Neither the Crown nor the universities deserve exclusive credit for university reform. In many cases the initiative for reform came from the universities themselves, as progressive faculty members came to realize that curriculum changes were essential. At the same time, the support of the Crown was necessary to compel more recalcitrant faculties and universities to put the proposed changes into effect. Thus, liberals within the universities created the new curricula, and the Crown imposed them on less progressive institutions. The Crown also used the reform movement for its own objectives of reducing clerical influence, standardizing higher education, and increasing royal control of the nation's intellectual and professional life.

The reform at the University of Salamanca was undoubtedly the most significant for Spain as a whole. Its traditional preeminence almost inevitably made reform there a model for universities elsewhere and probably helped to make reform acceptable to more conservative faculties. The oldest of Spanish universities also reveals the complexity of the relationship between school and state.

Progressive members of the Council of Castile such as the Conde de Campomanes began to dream of nationwide university reform during the early 1760s. In 1766, partly at the urging of liberal professors in the medical faculty at Salamanca, Campomanes ordered each faculty there to draw up a plan for reform. The medical professors eagerly complied, for although later events would prove them as concerned with professional status as any physician, they did not relate prestige to any particular curriculum. The educators strove to give the long-neglected subject of anatomy a paramount position and to base the new curriculum upon modern authors. By November their work was complete. Frustrated by the lack of activity elsewhere in the university, reformist professors sent Juan Martínez López, the professor of anatomy, to Madrid in order to present the new plan to Campomanes personally. He urged Campomanes to put pressure on the other faculties to get on with the work of reform.[12] The debate continued. Many professors worried at least as much over losing their privileges as over

12. AHN, Consejos, Leg. 5459, Expediente de Martínez López; Addy, *The Enlightenment in . . . Salamanca*, pp. 89–97.

the content of the innovations. Finally, in 1770, the entire university sent a complete proposal, including that of the medical faculty, to Madrid.[13]

Campomanes, who had his own ideas on educational reform, carefully studied the document, sought outside advice, and made numerous revisions. He completely reorganized the arts curriculum so that students would begin to specialize before receiving those degrees. As the medical faculty had recommended, future medical students would study mathematics and experimental physics, but Campomanes accepted the plan of the faculty of medicine in its original form.

The new plan, which was quite similar to that of the University of Cervera, would form the basis of Spanish medical education well into the nineteenth century. It sought to build a curriculum upon an author who had a logical approach with an emphasis on anatomy and experiment. He had to be up to date and widely respected throughout Europe. Fortunately, they chose the writings of Hermann Boerhaave, who, as we have seen, set the pattern for modern medical education throughout Europe.

According to the plan of studies created by the Salamancan physicians, the student would spend his first two years attending anatomical demonstrations and studying Boerhaave's *Institutiones medicae* to acquire a thorough grounding in general theory. For his last two years he would learn more practical material in Boerhaave's *Aphorismi de cognoscendis et curandis morbis.* The plan encouraged instructors to supplement these required texts with lectures from other classical and contemporary authors. It also created private academies in which every student would present a paper before his professors and fellow students. Finally, the plan called for the creation of an anatomical theater and a botanical garden.

Not everyone was satisfied with the change. The Protomedicato disapproved of the total reliance upon Boerhaave, finding him too "systematic," a valid criticism. Instead, the board suggested that the Salamanca faculty create its own course, using both classical and modern sources.[14] Yet it made better sense to follow the most respected contemporary author, for the eclectic type of course suggested by

13. For the text of the entire *Plan de estudios*, including Campomanes's revisions, see Addy, *The Enlightenment in . . . Salamanca*, pp. 244–366. On the reform, see also Mariano Peset Reig and José Luis Peset Reig, *El reformismo de Carlos III y la Universidad de Salamanca* (Salamanca, 1969).

14. AHN, Consejos, Leg. 5459, Exp. 6, Informe del Protomedicato, Aug. 21, 1769.

the board would probably have contained more errors than Boerhaave, to say nothing of the endless debates such a project would have engendered.

Nevertheless, the arguments for and against reform indicate a remarkable familiarity with modern authors on the part of professors and protomédicos alike. The authors of the reform had received their own formal education at Salamanca. Thus, it would appear that an archaic curriculum had never prevented some academics from becoming aware of the most recent scientific developments.

With the reform, however, modern medicine became the norm at Salamanca. Modern texts, frequent dissections, knowledgeable teachers, and better prepared students made a medical degree worthy of respect. Yet the plan was no panacea. Francisco Antonio de Zunzunegui, professor of anatomy, faced particularly serious problems. He constantly lacked enough money to buy needed instruments, and he never received the anatomical theater the plan had called for. Only after long delay was a dissector appointed to assist him. The hospital in Salamanca consistently refused to supply enough cadavers in spite of repeated royal edicts. At one point Zunzunegui had to use dogs. And he himself received less than one-third the salary of his colleagues.[15]

Under the tutelage of the enlightened ministers of Charles III, other universities soon followed suit. In 1769 the Crown decreed that a member of the Council of Castile was to serve as "director" of every Spanish university. His duty was to keep the Council informed of the university's academic and financial situation, and to encourage reform.[16] The following year the Council ordered all Spanish universities to draw up new curricula. The reactions varied. Many educators sincerely desired reform but were hesitant to make radical changes. Others opposed any change at all. As a general rule, Campomanes imposed the Salamancan curriculum on those universities that hesitated to reform themselves.

The other two universities that had a nationwide constituency, Alcalá and Valladolid, hesitated to follow Salamanca's lead. At the University of Alcalá, each faculty began to draw up a plan in response to the Council's order in 1770. The report of the faculty of medicine

15. AHN, Consejos, Leg. 5464, Exp. 14, Representación de Francisco Antonio Zunzunegui; Leg. 5460, Exp. 2, Representación del Claustro de Salamanca, Sept. 12, 1771; Leg. 5460, Exp. 39, Real provisión, July 21, 1772; Addy, *The Enlightenment in . . . Salamanca*, pp. 112–123.

16. *Nov. Rec.*, VIII, v, 1 and 2.

vaguely mentioned the value of Boerhaave, but was mostly concerned about low salaries.[17] The final statement of the full university *claustro* said little about medicine except to note the importance of anatomy. Moreover, declared the university, since most teachers and students "are imbued with the traditional system, it would be unwise to adopt a plan that would be totally alien to our methods."[18] Both statements angered Campomanes. Alcalá, he wrote, was completely decadent. Its traditional system was responsible for maintaining "prejudice, sophism, and superficiality in place of science and truth."[19] He ordered the faculty of medicine to draw up a more complete plan similar to that of Salamanca. Apparently that faculty did nothing. Campomanes then angrily imposed the complete Salamancan reforms upon Alcalá.[20] The university protested that the new plan was designed "to render obscure the true merit of ancient authorities [*sabios*]," but Campomanes allowed few concessions. Slowly and grudgingly Alcalá imposed the reforms, although by 1774 they were still not fully in effect.[21]

The University of Valladolid was even more recalcitrant. It proposed no change at all for its medical program, noting that Hippocrates and Galen were invaluable for their reliance on observation and experience. Campomanes imposed the Salamanca plan on Valladolid—the curriculum based on Boerhaave, a mandatory chair of anatomy, and periodic anatomical demonstrations open to the public.[22]

Perhaps the most ambitious—and earliest—reform occurred at the University of Seville, again as the result of the combined efforts of royal officials and progressive physicians. The reform-minded Seville Academy of Medicine had been attempting to introduce reforms within the university since the beginning of the century. In 1767 progressives both inside and outside the university dreamed of establishing a new institution of learning from the schools previously run by the suppressed Jesuits. A few months later they received invaluable support when Campomanes appointed Pablo de Olavide the new *intendente*, and entrusted him with the disposition of Jesuit wealth. Like Cam-

17. AHN, Consejos, Leg. 5430, Parte 1, núm. 13, Plan de la Facultad de Medicina, Jan 12, 1771.

18. *Ibid.*, Parte 1, núm. 13, Plan nuevo y méthodo de estudiar de todas las facultades, Feb. 28, 1771.

19. *Ibid.*, Parte 2, núm. 14, Repuesta fiscal, June 9, 1771.

20. *Ibid.*, Parte 1, núm. 13, Repuesta fiscal, Nov. 13, 1772.

21. AHN, Consejos, Leg. 5431, Exp. 3, Testimonial de Dr. Josef Pinilla, May 2, 1774; Real pragmática, Dec. 11, 1772, in *Cartulario*, pp. 565–569.

22. Real cédula, June 21, 1771, in *Cartulario*, pp. 515–519; Ajo González, *Historia de las universidades*, V, 216–219.

pomanes, though more radical, Olavide considered himself an ilustrado and was dedicated to modernizing Spanish life.

Olavide, working closely with liberals on the university faculty, decided to completely overhaul the university and then attach the Jesuit schools to a thoroughly modern institution. Their plan called for the elimination of private colleges, autonomy from the state, and, most important of all, freedom from what Olavide called the antiquated Scholastic spirit that had so permeated education that graduates were unprepared to practice their profession.[23]

Their proposed curriculum for the faculty of medicine resembled that of Salamanca in its reliance on Boerhaave, but it was more extensive. The five-year program proceeded logically from the natural sciences to anatomy and physiology to therapeutics, pharmacy, and practice. Both traditional and modern authors were recommended as texts. Olavide significantly observed that surgery did not belong in a university but should be taught in special schools or hospitals.[24]

The Council of Castile was impressed with the Olavide plan, but it hesitated to approve it because of the cost. Finally, in 1769, the Council endorsed the plan in principle and, making some changes that brought it more in line with the Salamancan reform, ordered its implementation.[25] Seville, with Valencia, would remain a center of medical education for the rest of the century.

As other universities fell into line, a notable similarity existed among the various plans. Most resembled Salamanca. Campomanes had accomplished his objective of combining reform with greater uniformity and royal control. Meanwhile, the Council issued numerous decrees to further standardize higher education. The surgical colleges would later have to fit into the comprehensive framework set up for medicine. In 1770, for example, the Council decreed that all medical students had to study logic, metaphysics, arithmetic, algebra, geometry, and experimental physics before turning to medicine itself. At the same time the Council made a four-year medical course mandatory and established a

23. Pablo de Olavide, *Plan de estudios para la Universidad de Sevilla*, with intro. by Francisco Aguilar Piñal (Barcelona, 1969), pp. 79–88. On the Seville reforms, see also Marcelin Defourneaux, *Pablo de Olavide, el afrancesado*, trans. Manuel Martínez Camaro (Mexico City, 1965); Francisco Aguilar Piñal, *La Universidad de Seville en el siglo XVIII: Estudio sobre la primera reforma universitaria moderna* (Seville, 1969), pp. 133–262.

24. Olavide, *Plan*, pp. 130–138. It is unclear if Salamanca influenced Seville or vice versa, since progressives everywhere were thinking along the same lines.

25. Jovellanos, *Informe, . . . sobre medicina*; Aguilar Piñal, *La Universidad de Sevilla*, pp. 252–262; Defourneaux, *Pablo de Olavide*, pp. 90–92.

required number of hours per course. In other areas the Council standardized the procedures for examinations and faculty appointments, mandated that all degrees be accepted by any university, and ordered all notices of faculty vacancies to be posted in every university so that more candidates would apply for the positions. On occasion the Council also eliminated university programs for which there was insufficient staff.[26]

Although the Council of Castile constantly endeavored to establish the high standards set forth in the individual plans throughout Spain, it occasionally made concessions to tradition. A 1777 decree setting forth the obligations of professors of anatomy is a case in point.[27] It required the professor to illustrate his lectures with "good engravings and prepared exhibits of skeletons and artificial bodies," and to hold periodic dissections. However, recognizing the problems of obtaining human cadavers, the Council required their dissection only "when conditions permit." Moreover, the plans imposed on individual universities had specified the texts of Martín Martínez, the Spanish anatomist, or Lorenz Heister.[28] The 1777 decree, however, merely required the professor to use Hippocrates, Galen, Vesalius, and "recent authors." Perhaps conservative opposition had forced the Council to tread more carefully by 1777. Or perhaps its conservative president, Manual Ventura Figueroa (1773–1783), was less inclined to press for change.

In spite of some setbacks university reform culminated in a 1786 *cédula* (decree) that once and for all unified every aspect of university education.[29] Using Salamanca as a model, it described in detail the curricula, academic year, requirements for matriculation and degrees, and procedures for the *oposición*, or contest for an academic chair, for every university in Spain. Henceforth, the "more useful" modern philosophy would be taught in place of that "popularly called Scholasticism." Universities were not to accept arts degrees earned in private colleges without an additional examination.

26. AHN, Universidades, Leg. 42, Edicto del Real Consejo, Oct. 16, 1771; Real cédula, Jan. 24, 1770, and Real pragmática, July 9, 1770, in *Cartulario*, pp. 472 and 481, respectively; *Nov. Rec.*, VII, vii, 7.

27. Real provisión, 1777, quoted in Sánchez Granjel, *Anatomía española*, p. 16.

28. Such was the case at Alcalá, Valladolid, Granada, and Santiago, among others.

29. AHN, Consejos, Leg. 5444, Exp. 15, Parte 3, Real Cédula . . . por la qual se manda que en todas las Universidades de estos Reynos . . . se observe en ellas lo dispuesto y establecido para la de Salamanca en quanto a la matrícula de Estudiantes, su asistencia a Cátedras, exercicios de Academias, oposiciones a Cátedras, exámenes para el pase de unas a otras . . . , Jan. 22, 1786, and accompanying memorandum of Floridablanca, Nov. 18, 1785.

Surgery posed special problems in establishing reform, standardization, and royal control in the universities. Students were few; chairs of surgery were often vacant. Salamanca used a text of Guido Guidi, a a fourteenth-century French surgeon.[30] However, while university surgery had grown more and more decadent, new institutions had arisen. By 1770 there were outstanding schools of surgery in Cádiz and Barcelona, plans for another in Madrid, and countless semiautonomous colleges and academies. As a result, the reformers of university surgery took into account the efforts to reform the profession as a whole. They sought to bring sense and order into the whole structure of chaotic, contradictory regulations and institutions that dominated the science.

In order to combat both decadence and confusion, Campomanes decided to reform university surgery where possible and to abolish it where it was beyond hope or where it duplicated the efforts of independent surgical colleges. In 1768 he suppressed the chairs of both surgery and anatomy at the University of Cervera, since similar chairs existed in the Barcelona college. Even medical students from Cervera were to study anatomy for a year at Barcelona.[31] Three years later, noting that one chair was insufficient for training surgeons anyway, he suppressed the chair of surgery at Alcalá since plans existed for a similar college in Madrid.[32]

Only the progressive medical faculty at Salamanca was able to retain its surgical program. Its reform proposals had included a four-year course for Latin surgeons, to consist of two years of anatomy and Boerhaave's *Instituciones* (identical to the first two years in medicine), followed by two years of surgery and more anatomy. *Quirurgía repurgata* by Johann Gorter, a Dutch surgeon and student of Boerhaave, was chosen as the text for surgery.[33]

Pleased with the proposal, though still unwilling to rely completely on advice from a university, Campomanes decided to consult the College of San Fernando, the controversial surgical academy founded by Ferdinand VI. The college responded with a lengthy statement.[34] It praised the Salamancan reformers for their concern, but added that

30. Plan de Medicina, 1766.

31. AGS, Gracia y Justicia, Leg. 405 (992), *Plan de Estudios de Medicina para la Universidad de Cervera* (Madrid, 1784). The *Plan* quoted the cédula of Dec. 15, 1768, that made the change.

32. AHN, Consejos, Leg. 5430, Parte 2, Exp. 14, Repuesta fiscal, June 9, 1771.

33. *Plan general de Salamanca* (1771), in Addy, *The Enlightenment in . . . Salamanca*, p. 323.

34. AHN, Consejos, Leg. 5459, Exp. 6, Informe del Colegio de San Fernando de Cirujanos de Madrid, June 23, 1767.

as physicians they lacked the knowledge and experience to teach surgery competently. Indeed, it continued, "the lack of knowledge of physicians, and the unjustified superiority they presume to possess over surgeons, are the reason Spanish surgery has reached its present decadence." The Salamancan plan was far too theoretical, and Gorter was of dubious value for beginners. Moreover, most practicing surgeons were not university-educated anyway. The real solution, concluded the report, was to remove all surgical education from the university and to establish special schools of surgery independent of both the universities and the Protomedicato.

Campomanes decided to approve the plan submitted by the Salamancan professors, but he took steps to guarantee the existing surgical schools equal status with that university. A royal edict ordered Salamanca to post notices for an oposición for anatomical dissector, not only in all major universities, as was customary, but also in the two surgical colleges.[35]

Despite all problems, however, by 1780 medical education in Spanish universities was among the best available in Europe. Reforms had brought about a uniform curriculum based on modern authors. Anatomy had a dominant position. Medical students had a good background in the natural sciences.[36] Yet legislated reforms were not able to solve all the ills that plagued medicine. Physicians still mistrusted surgeons; the Salamancan faculty was outraged at the thought that the anatomical dissector, trained at Cádiz, might become the professor of anatomy.[37] Student enrollment remained very small. By 1785 Salamanca had only 21 students studying medicine compared with 653 studying theology and 527 studying law and canon law. Surprisingly, however, 22 students were studying Latin surgery. In the other two major universities together (Alcalá and Valladolid) there were 45 students enrolled in medicine, 384 in theology, and 646 in law and canon law.[38]

Filling the professorships also remained a problem. During the 1780s the University of Salamanca had trouble filling both the chair of anat-

35. AHN, Consejos, Leg. 5462, Exp. 39, Real provisión, July 21, 1772.

36. AHN, Consejos, Leg. 5444, Exp. 1, Informes, 1796. This expediente contains an informe from every Spanish university describing its curricula, textbooks, degree requirements, and the like.

37. AHN, Consejos, Leg. 5465, Exp. 21, Representación de Isidro Alonso del Campal, Sept. 5, 1786.

38. *Guía histórica de las universidades, colegios, academias y demás cuerpos literarios de España y América* (Madrid, 1786), pp. 26–85.

omy and the chair of surgery.[39] At Alcalá even the traditional chairs of medicine were often vacant. During the 1770s, also at Alcalá, as many as thirty-three men applied for a vacant chair of canons and as many as forty for a chair of theology. When chairs of medicine became vacant, however, there were never more than three applicants. Indeed, in the case of one chair the very same men turned down the first time were the only applicants when the chair again became vacant. Filling the chair of anatomy was even more difficult, for on two separate occasions a vacancy was announced and only one man applied. Moreover, the oposición was a poor test of ability since it often seemed more a test of memory than of understanding.[40] Thus, many of the old problems remained.

Although academic reform had vastly improved the quality of medical education in the universities, it had not solved the larger problems facing the profession. In addition, the very process of modernization had cost the universities much of their traditional autonomy, despite the significant contributions of academics themselves. The Crown not only compelled recalcitrant faculties to reform but looked upon the universities as just one of many approaches to medical progress. By the 1780s the Council of Castile was clearly contemplating national approaches to medical reform. The age of individual institutional initiative was past. During the 1790s the progressive faculty of medicine at Salamanca submitted plans for further reform. The Council of Castile, which by then was formulating its own plans for nationwide reform, simply ignored them.[41] Thus, by the time Charles III died in 1788, Madrid clearly exercised complete dominion over the training and practice of doctors.

Indeed, most reformers had little hope for the universities. Rather than attempt to revive what they regarded as lethargic institutions burdened by age-old traditions and established structures, they looked to the creation of new institutions of learning directed by educators under royal supervision. As a result, the eighteenth century witnessed the creation of countless new royal academies and colleges created through the efforts of a few individuals.

39. AHN, Consejos, Leg. 5465, Exp. 21, Representación de Isidro Alonso del Campal, Sept. 5, 1786.

40. AHN, Universidades, Leg. 42, Orden del Consejo, Sept. 25, 1784; AHN, Consejos, Leg. 5430, Parte 2, Expedientes 9–22; Leg. 5431, Expedientes 3, 31, 53. (These *legajos* contain full records of all oposiciones at Alcalá.)

41. See Addy, *The Enlightenment in . . . Salamanca*, pp. 175–177, 204.

Although the complete renovation of higher education had no counterpart outside of Spain, the establishment of new institutions dedicated to education and research occurred throughout Europe. In England hospitals began anatomical demonstrations and clinical training, while individual practitioners offered private classes in medicine and surgery. French hospitals and private instructors offered similar training, and the Crown endowed chairs in medicine and the natural sciences in a variety of institutions. In 1731 the French Crown approved the establishment of a Royal Academy of Surgery.[42]

Alternatives to the universities were particularly important in the reform of surgery, for in no other traditional discipline had higher education failed so dismally. Long before the overhaul of university medicine, reformers began to move in two directions. The first was informal hospital training. As early as the reign of Philip V leading surgeons and anatomists began offering instruction in hospitals. Later they formed academies to provide a means of exchanging information on new discoveries and techniques. These initial steps were relatively easy to put into effect, for they offered no direct challenge to existing licensing and degree-granting institutions. The second major step was the founding of formal schools of surgery with the authority to set standards and grant licenses. Endowed chairs in hospitals and colleges would not only raise educational standards but also provide surgeons with the hope of winning dignified positions with a comfortable income. If surgery were ever to attract promising young men, it had to offer more than poverty and public scorn.[43]

Since the sixteenth century hospitals had provided some future physicians and surgeons with the years of practice required by the Protomedicato. Until the eighteenth century, however, most *practicantes* merely performed menial tasks such as serving patients their meals. Philip V took the first step to make this internship more valuable by endowing a chair of anatomy in 1701. Public lectures began in 1707.[44] In 1747, Ferdinand VI issued new regulations for the practicantes at the Hospital General.[45] The ordinances recognized that

42. Toby Gelfand, "The 'Paris Manner' of Dissection: Student Anatomical Dissection in Early Eighteenth-Century Paris," *Bulletin of the History of Medicine*, XLVI (1972), 112 ff.; Gelfand, "From Guild to Profession," p. 127; Coury, "The Teaching of Medicine in France," pp. 141–147.

43. This problem is discussed in the *Correo de Madrid, o de los Ciegos*, I (June 9, 1787), 283–284.

44. Sánchez Granjel, *Anatomía española*, pp. 20–21.

45. Archivo de la Diputación Provincial de Madrid (hereinafter cited as ADP),

"hospitals are the best schools for true medical practice" and also required the practicantes to attend dissections and lectures. The professor of anatomy was to hold separate lectures for the public at large.

The new regulations also provided for eight practicantes in surgery. An applicant for the position had only to show he had led a good life, was truly dedicated, and that his parents had never held an infamous occupation. He apparently did not have to meet the usual requirements of legitimate birth in an old Christian family ("limpieza de sangre"). Once accepted, the practicante would spend three years assisting the regular surgeons in their rounds and attending classes in anatomy, surgical operations, and dressing wounds. Though still a romance surgeon, the "graduate" was obviously far better trained than most.

By the middle of the eighteenth century there had arisen a small number of well-educated, highly skilled surgeons. Some had taught themselves; others had studied under expert professors or in new hospital programs. The new professionals were extremely scornful of the mass of untrained, ignorant surgeons who dominated the profession. In order to raise standards and to bring this small elite together in a formal body, Thomas Duchesnay Desprez, First Surgeon of Ferdinand VI, urged his monarch to establish a special academy. Having studied in Paris himself, he argued that only by imitating the successful academies there could Spanish anatomy and surgery ever become respectable. In 1747 the Crown complied with the creation of the Surgical College of San Fernando of Madrid.[46]

Originally the college was a professional association, not a school. Members described their most recent accomplishments in formal lectures and notified each other of impending experiments. The college kept records and publicized the latest scientific advances made in Spain and abroad. Members forswore such unsavory, though common, procedures as castration for intestinal malignancies.

The college was undoubtedly successful in disseminating the latest knowledge and techniques, but its members wanted to move beyond their own narrow circle and work to reform the profession as a whole. Here, as described in the previous chapter, the college ran head-on into the opposition of the Protomedicato and the Confradía of San Cosme

Leg. 118, Borrador de las Ordenanzas para el gobierno de los Hospitales Generales y Pasión de Madrid, 1747.

46. AGS, Secretaría de Hacienda, Leg. 549, Estatutos del Real Colegio de Profesores Cirujanos de Madrid, 1747.

and San Damian. The Protomedicato, frowning upon the pretensions of mere surgeons, resisted the attack on its prerogatives. The practicing surgeons and barbers of the Confradía resented the small coterie with highly paid government positions who seemed determined to monopolize the profession. In 1749 the college lost the right to license its own members. Undaunted, the college proceeded to propose a complete program of studies for future surgeons. Although the Council of Castile took no direct action, the college seized every opportunity over the next few years to argue the need of an independent school of surgery. Its petitions were no doubt instrumental in the eventual founding of San Carlos. Meanwhile, the college continued to hold lectures, offer instruction in surgery and anatomy, send students abroad for study, and, in general, fight for the highest standards in the profession.[47]

The Hospital General professors and the faculty of the College of San Fernando worked closely together. In 1760 Juan Gámez, a former practicante who would himself win its chair of anatomy, wrote a new set of ordinances for the Hospital General.[48] First Gámez extended the anatomy course for physicians over three years. The first year would cover general anatomical principles and the study of bones and muscles; the second year, the study of arteries, glands, and nerves; and the third year, the organs and reproductive system. Thus, anatomy was far more thorough and better organized for the practicantes than for university students even after the reforms. Indeed, the future physician, restricted by law to internal medicine, quite likely learned more anatomy than he could realistically expect to use. Gámez outlined a similarly detailed program in surgery. The practicante would attend the anatomy lessons during the fall, though not those concerning glands, the preserve of internal medicine; he would also receive special lessons in surgery that were cycled over a three-year period.

Despite the importance Gámez gave to anatomy, he emphasized that the day-to-day practice of the practicante was the essence of his hospital experience. Unfortunately, this experience was restricted to very few young men; no more than about twenty-five practicantes ever served at any one time.[49]

47. Informe de Colegio de Cirujanos de Madrid, 1753, in Consulta sobre cirugía.

48. ADP, Leg. 118, *Constituciones y Ordenanzas para el gobierno de los Reales Hospitales General, y de la Pasión de Madrid* (Madrid, 1760). Alvarez-Sierra, *Historia de la cirugía española*, p. 237, attributes the *ordenanzas* to Gámez.

49. AGS, Gracia y Justicia, Leg. 404 (989), Representación de Juan Gámez, Dec. 23, 1771.

The progressive surgeons must have been enthusiastic over the new program. Yet a hospital on its own could have but limited effect. Few surgeons were exposed to the new training; those who participated did so at their own choice and received no special certification for doing so. Licensing standards remained unchanged. As a result, the progressive surgeons were convinced that only when the new brand of surgical education became the norm for the entire profession would surgery as a whole benefit. So once again the reforming surgeons pleaded for a full-scale school of surgery. In 1771 Campomanes agreed.[50]

By 1770 a genuine school of surgery was not a utopian idea. In past years the Crown had established numerous teaching academies and colleges in other disciplines. More than one thousand students were studying in Madrid alone. The Conde de Aranda, president of the Council of Castile, had visions of a grand university in Madrid to teach all things that existing universities ignored.[51] Moreover, two schools of surgery already existed in Cádiz and Barcelona. Every petition for a Madrid school had referred to these schools as possible models.

Considering the jealousy with which the universities, guilds, and the Protomedicato traditionally guarded their privileges, two factors had made possible the establishment of the two schools of surgery. First was the fact that both schools were under control of the Spanish military. Medicine in the army and navy had long been separate from civilian practice, and often it was more advanced. Both branches of the service had hospitals under their control. The Cádiz college, for example, was attached to the Royal Hospital of the Navy there, which had offered anatomical instruction since 1728.[52] Military medicine often required special skills. Accordingly, since students of both schools were destined to become army or naval surgeons, neither school posed an immediate threat to the civilian medical establishment.

The second factor seems to have been the indomitable personality of the schools' founder, Pedro Virgili, (1699–1776), and the influential friends he made at court. Virgili was raised in a small Catalonian town in a family of limited means. As a youth he assisted the local physician, a dedicated man who occasionally practiced dissections on his own.

50. Informe de Josef Fernández, 1764; Dictamen de Pedro Perchet y Pedro Virgili, July 10, 1768; Repuesta fiscal, Oct. 18, 1771, all in Consulta sobre Cirugía.

51. La Fuente, *Historia de las universidades*, IV, 168–175.

52. Sánchez Granjel, *Anatomía española*, pp. 25–26. This account of the founding of the Cádiz school is based on Ferrer, *Colegio de Cádiz*, pp. 1–108; García del Real, *Historia de la medicina en España*, pp. 444–447; La Fuente, *Historia de las universidades*, IV, 179–180; Hernández Morejón, *Historia bibliográfica*, III, 341–346.

Eager to learn more of anatomy, young Virgili journeyed to Montpellier, where he studied surgery and anatomy, and then to Paris, where he met some of the most renowned surgeons of his day. Upon his return, he joined the army as a surgeon. His reputation grew rapidly as he performed such complicated operations for his day as a tracheotomy. While near Gibraltar Virgili met another celebrated surgeon, Juan de Lacomba. Lacomba, whose son would play an important role at San Carlos, had established the anatomy classes at the Cádiz naval hospital. In the late 1720s Virgili, at the behest of his friend, became a naval surgeon and joined the hospital staff. His friendship with Lacomba would serve him well, for Lacomba introduced Virgili to Zenón de Somodevilla, the Marqués de la Ensenada. Ensenada, secretary of the treasury, war, the navy, and the Indies under Ferdinand VI, was devoting much of his time to modernizing the Spanish military. Improved medical facilities were to be one part of this reform.

In May 1748 Virgili sent Ensenada a detailed proposal for a school of surgery. He argued that such a school would help solve the serious shortage of naval surgeons. The school would combine classroom and clinic. It would have full-time teachers and formal examinations. By locating it in the Cádiz hospital, students would also receive first-hand experience. In order to matriculate, according to Virgili's proposal, a young man would have to be able to read, write, and do simple arithmetic. He would also have to prove he was "of a good family free of bad lineage, behavior, and tendencies."[53] Since the requirement of limpieza de sangre was customary for admission to universities, the new school would have been little respected had it not also imposed it.

At the urging of Ensenada, the Crown accepted Virgili's proposal as part of a program of new schools for naval personnel. The statutes, issued in November 1748, established a three-year course that emphasized anatomy and practical experience.[54] A few weeks later Lacomba died, and Virgili became chief surgeon of the navy and director of the new college.

During the next decade both Virgili and the school prospered. Virgili received a title in 1753, and was named First Surgeon of the Royal Chamber in 1758, after which he spent most of his time in

53. "Hijos de buenos padres, limpios de mala raza, costumbres e inclinaciones." Memorial de Pedro Virgili, May 29, 1748, quoted in full in Ferrer, *Colegio de Cádiz*, pp. 44–51.

54. Estatutos del Real Colegio de Cirugía de Cádiz, Nov. 18, 1748, quoted in full in Ferrer, *ibid.*, pp. 56–60.

Madrid. The college first opened its doors in 1750. Before long it possessed its own building, an anatomical theater, a library, and a small botanical garden. Occasionally the college sent its more promising graduates to Paris, Montpellier, Leyden, and Bologna for additional study. Meanwhile, the program was expanded to four years, and students were offered the humanities courses necessary for a bachelor of arts degree. In 1757, after a protracted struggle with the Protomedicato, Virgili won for the school the right to license all its graduates as Latin surgeons without additional examination. No university ever acquired this privilege.

The school also served as a focal point for scientific activity. Some of the century's most notable scientists, including Jorge Juan and Antonio de Ulloa, came to Cádiz to observe the progress there. Frequent formal exercises (*actos*) provided professors, students, and outside scientists an opportunity to present their latest research. Many graduates of the school would later become famous in their own right.

Stimulated by the success of the Cádiz school, Virgili next began to agitate for a similar school for army surgeons in his native Catalonia.[55] Ferdinand VI approved the idea in 1758, and Charles III approved its statutes in 1760. Four years later the school opened its doors to some fifty students in a Barcelona hospital. It, too, had a distinguished faculty, an anatomical theater, and its own building.

The inauguration of the Barcelona college was more than the opening of a school for army surgeons. For Diego Velasco, who gave the inaugural address, the college marked the end of an era. No longer would Spaniards have to rely on ignorant, untrained surgeons who knew nothing of science. No longer would harmful treatments cause soldiers to die needlessly from battle wounds. No longer would the nation have to rely on foreigners for competent medical care.[56]

The inauguration also marked an important step in the government's efforts to standardize the surgical colleges and to separate them from existing institutions. A few months preceding the opening ceremonies the Crown approved statutes written by Pedro Virgili and Pedro Perchet, also a Surgeon of the Royal Chamber, that established iden-

55. The account of the Barcelona school is based on García del Real, *Historia de la medicina en España*, pp. 447–448; Sánchez Granjel, *Anatomía española*, p. 27; La Fuente, *Historia de las universidades*, IV, 178–181; Hernández Morejón, *Historia bibliográfica*, III, 341–346.

56. Diego Velasco, "Discurso inaugural," quoted in García del Real, *Historia de la medicina en España*, pp. 442–443, n. 1.

tical curricula at both schools.[57] The new statutes defined five professorships: physiology and pathology, osteology (the study of bones), surgical operations, anatomy, and therapeutics, which included bleeding, cauterizing, application of bandages, and other common procedures. The professors of anatomy and surgery were to illustrate their lessons on cadavers. Thus, for the first time medical education was organized not by authors but according to the logical divisions of the science.

Virgili's ordinances were also something of a declaration of independence for surgery, at least in Catalonia, where traditional institutions had been under attack since the War of the Spanish Succession. The statutes declared that graduates of the school should be treated in all respects just as if they had graduated from a university. They could practice anywhere in Spain without an additional license. Moreover, the statutes placed all colleges and guilds of surgeons in Catalonia under the new school. Henceforth, the Barcelona College of Surgery, not the Protomedicato or the guilds, would grant all licenses to practice surgery there. In order to become a master surgeon, that is, one who could perform all procedures and train others, one had to have either graduated from the school or have had six years of experience in the art, two as an apprentice under a licensed master. The minimum age was twenty-two, although sons of master surgeons could be licensed at twenty years because they "had applied themselves to surgery since childhood."

Efforts to reform the training of Spanish surgeons were not restricted to the Iberian peninsula. In 1767, in response to the petitions of Mexican surgeons and the viceroy of New Spain, the Crown established chairs of anatomy and surgery in Mexico City in imitation of the schools in Cádiz and Barcelona. During the next decade Mexican surgeons, supported by the viceroy, urged that the hospital instruction be expanded into a complete school, independent from the university and the Protomedicato. In 1783 the Crown agreed.[58]

57. *Estatutos . . . que S.M. manda observar a los Colegios, y Comunidades de Cirujanos, establecidos en Barcelona, Cádiz, y en todo el Principado de Cataluña* (Madrid, 1764). A copy exists in the library of the Academia de Medicina, Madrid.

58. Reales cédulas, May 20, 1768, and July 14, 1783, in Romulo Velasco Ceballos, *La cirugía mexicana en el siglo XVIII* (Mexico City, 1946), pp. 35–36, 103–108.

The case of surgery would seem to suggest that the scientific and educational reforms of the eighteenth century occurred in similar fashion throughout the Spanish Empire. Peninsular and American surgeons had strikingly similar objectives for modernizing education and restructuring the profession. Both relied on royal support to overcome the established interests of the Protomedicato and the universities. Un-

Within Spain, there existed two colleges of surgery that provided a thoroughly modern education even before the first reforms occurred in the universities. Here all the innovations mentioned at the beginning of this chapter were already in effect—modern texts, a rational division of the subject, emphasis on anatomy, clinical experience. In Catalonia the high standards of the colleges were imposed on the entire profession. To be sure, it was but a start. Graduates of the schools were few in number; most of them would serve in the armed forces. The Protomedicato, the universities, and the guilds were still as powerful as ever in most of Spain. Nevertheless, by the 1760s there was a strong movement toward radical innovations among reformist elements both in the government and in the profession itself. The hospital instruction and, above all, the colleges in Cádiz and Barcelona had shown what such innovation could accomplish.

fortunately, since most research has concentrated on one area or the other, more research on the transfer of culture is warranted before final conclusions can be made.

CHAPTER IV

# THE ESTABLISHMENT OF THE COLLEGE OF SAN CARLOS

On October 1, 1787, a well-dressed assemblage gathered in the basement of the Hospital General of Madrid, near the Gate of Atocha on the outskirts of the city. The building had a long history, even by 1787. Some of Spain's most renowned physicians and surgeons had given classes and carried on experiments within its walls. Yet the hospital wards were dirty, overcrowded, and decidedly unsanitary. Excessive heat and putrid odors were everywhere. Several patients were often crowded into one bed. Relatively healthy patients were thrown in with those who were near death or suffering from contagious diseases. It was not unknown for a patient to leave the hospital in worse condition than when he had entered. A new addition had been constructed in the early 1780s, but it had not alleviated the shortage of beds or the inescapable stench.[1]

The notables of Madrid had not come to discuss the unhealthy conditions in the wards. Rather, they had come together to celebrate the formal opening of the Royal College of Surgery of San Carlos in Madrid. For decades plans for such a college had been proposed, studied, criticized, revised, and finally, in 1780, approved. Amid the excitement of it all, between the formal speeches and learned dissertations, perhaps no one was bothered by the fact that the inauguration of such a promising institution was taking place in the basement. The new building that had been promised to the school was not yet completed.[2]

The ceremonies that took place that Monday morning had been planned down to the last detail. At the request of the school's director, Antonio Gimbernat, two members of the Council of Castile presided.[3]

1. Pérez de Escobar, *Medicina patria*, 42–43.

2. AHN, Consejos, Leg. 1035, Exp. 1, Parte 1, Aviso del Consejo, May 2, 1787.

3. The two were Rodrigo de la Torre Marín and Pablo Ferrándiz Bendicho. The plans for the inaugural ceremonies are summarized in AHN, Consejos, Leg. 1035, Exp. 1, Parte 1, Aviso del Consejo, Sept. 27, 1787. The ceremonies themselves are described

A private ceremony took place first. The two ministers formally gave possession of the school to Gimbernat and installed the professors in their chairs. A short tour of the facilities followed—the board room, the library, the anatomical theater, the small museum, the laboratory, and the classrooms. Then Rodrigo de Torre Marín, one of the two ministers, gave a short address. The new school, he declared, would restore "the dying art of surgery" to its rightful position.

At eleven o'clock the doors opened. A crowd of doctors, government officials, and hospital personnel flocked in for the public ceremony. Antonio Gimbernat spoke briefly of the great hopes he had for the new school. He was especially proud of its independence from other medical bodies. He then proceeded to deliver his formal address, a learned lecture on the correct use of sutures. The address was later to be deposited in the school's archives. Regular classes would begin the next day.

For Antonio Gimbernat, Pedro Custodio Gutiérrez, the president of the school, and countless other dedicated men, that inaugural ceremony was the culmination of years of work. Now their dream was a reality. San Carlos had an adequate physical plant, a dedicated faculty, a supply of instruments, an endowment, and a few students. The day had personal meaning to Gimbernat, too, for his son Carlos had been admitted as the first resident student of the school on a full scholarship.[4]

The long, difficult road that led to that inaugural day in 1787 tells as much about the personalities and procedures of the government of Charles III as it does about surgery. Caution and prudence were the principal hallmarks of Spanish administration. Few actions were taken without endless consultation in every quarter. Although the pages and pages of proposals and criticisms on San Carlos no doubt contributed much to its ultimate success, one cannot but sympathize with the frustrations the college's advocates must have felt during the interminable delays.

The earliest dreams of an autonomous school of surgery in Madrid originated in the College of San Fernando, the research institute founded by Ferdinand VI in 1748. In it Madrid's new breed of well-trained, highly dedicated surgeons had for the first time an official

---

in AHN, Consejos, Leg. 3514, Exp. 17, Parte 6, Testamento de Torre Marín y Ferrándiz, n.d., which contains the texts of the speeches, and in the *Gaceta de Madrid*, Oct. 19, 1787, p. 707.

4. AHN, Consejos, Leg. 1035, Exp. 1, Parte 1, Real orden, Sept. 3, 1787.

organization through which they could lobby for reform. As we have seen, the new college immediately challenged the Protomedicato and the Confradía of San Cosme and San Damian. Rivalry between these traditional institutions and the reformers would hinder real progress for decades to come.

The college first proposed formal surgical instruction in 1753 as part of an effort to counter the pretensions of the confraternity.[5] Its plan consisted of classes based on the various fields of medicine, not on specific authors, as was then customary. Anatomy, physiology, and pathology would form the basic curriculum. At this point the efforts of the college were directed toward providing romance surgeons with a theoretical background.

This original proposal also called for autonomy from the Protomedicato, creating an issue that would continue to plague all future deliberations over the school. The Protomedicato, it argued, was incompetent, ignorant of modern surgery, and a hindrance to reform. The college pointed to independent schools in Paris and London and to the new school in Cádiz as examples of what autonomy could accomplish.

Unfortunately, nothing came of the proposal. It was apparently lost in the intricacies of the dispute between the college and the confraternity, but its proponents did not give up. In 1764 they once again used an unrelated quarrel to put forth their plan.

This time Campomanes had initiated an attack on the Protomedicato. It seems he had come across an edict of the Protomedicato requiring physicians to perform bloodlettings and purges in medical cases. It was a clear case of the physicians' abusing their authority in order to restrict surgeons still further. In answer to his angry protest, the Protomedicato explained that surgeons could attend cases that required *only* the "application of hands."[6] Still dissatisfied, Campomanes sought the advice of the College of San Fernando. Joseph Fernández, dissector of the college, responded that such abuses were inevitable as long as surgery was subordinate to medicine. He echoed the previous plea for an autonomous college similar to those in Cádiz and Barcelona, and added that Pedro Virgili had endorsed the original proposal.[7]

In 1767 the college once again endorsed the idea of a school of

5. Informe del Colegio de San Fernando, 1753, in Consulta sobre cirugía.

6. Aviso de Campomanes, 1764, and Informe del Protomedicato, 1764, in Consulta sobre cirugía.

7. Informe de Josef Fernández, 1764, in Consulta sobre cirugía.

surgery when the Council asked it to comment on the reform proposal of the Salamancan faculty of medicine. This time Fernández urged that university chairs of surgery be transferred to such a school. He added that Madrid would have had "the methods of education [used] in the schools of Paris" by now if only "the Protomedicato had not hindered their progress."[8]

Thus, by 1768 the movement for reforming surgical education entailed two distinct significant innovations: the establishment of an autonomous college of surgery, and self-government for the surgical profession outside the jurisdiction of the Protomedicato. Although the two reforms were clearly related in the eyes of their proponents, the issue of autonomy would form a major barrier to a college of surgery for years to come. By demanding autonomy, the reformers provoked the opposition of the powerful Royal Protomedicato, which otherwise might well have supported a surgical college.

The Council of Castile, on the other hand, was predisposed to look favorably upon proposals that challenged traditional authorities not under its direct jurisdiction. Imbued, too, with the spirit of reform, it turned its full attention to the training of surgeons in 1769. Once again, a minor question initiated discussion. The anatomical demonstrator at the Hospital General at the time was Pedro Custodio Gutiérrez, who later became president of the College of San Carlos. Because he had been educated in Paris, the hospital petitioned that he be named First Surgeon in spite of the carefully defined seniority system in its statutes. Though impressed with the young anatomist's credentials, the Council denied the petition. The Council did order, however, that Custodio Gutiérrez head a committee within the hospital to draw up a new plan for training surgeons there.[9]

After several minor jurisdictional disputes Custodio Gutiérrez set to work. In early spring the hospital forwarded his plan, slightly revised, to the Crown.[10] The problem in the eyes of the young surgeon

8. AHN, Consejos, Leg. 5459, Exp. 6, Informe del Colegio de San Fernando, June 23, 1767.

9. Summarized in AGS, Secretaría de Hacienda, Leg. 949, Copia del expediente del nuevo Colegio de Cirugía de Madrid, división en las tres facultades. . . , y demás incidencias, March 5, 1784 (hereinafter cited as Expediente del nuevo Colegio). This is a lengthy narrative and summary of events between 1768 and 1784 sent to the Protomedicato. An examination of many of the paraphrased documents testifies to the veracity of the summary.

10. AGS, Gracia y Justicia, Leg. 404 (989). Representación de Pedro Custodio Gutiérrez, n.d. His proposed statutes are included. Though this document is undated, other evidence clearly indicates that this is his 1768 proposal.

was threefold: Latin surgeons were too few, romance surgeons were too ignorant, and the examinations of the Protomedicato were ludicrous rituals whose only purpose was to collect money. His solution was a Madrid college that would train surgeons, license all nonphysicians, and hold lectures and seminars. To be admitted, students would merely have to prove their limpieza de sangre. There would be five professors, each of whom would specialize in one branch of medicine. He added that all professors would have to be proficient in Latin and another foreign language, since so few texts were available in Spanish.

Custodio Gutiérrez, who was more interested in the regulation of surgery than in teaching it, went on to propose a complex reorganization of the profession. Henceforth, surgery would be divided into First Class surgeons (arts degree, some university medicine, classroom surgery, and practice), Second Class surgeons (some Latin, six years of practice), Third Class surgeons (less practice, prohibited from performing operations), hernia specialists, oculists, midwives, and dentists. The proposed college, not the Protomedicato, would hold examinations and grant licenses for all practitioners in these fields whether or not they had attended the school. His proposed ordinances carefully described the nature of the examination for each class. The examination for First Class surgeon would extend over nine days. In a final appeal to the pocketbook, Custodio Gutiérrez showed how licensing fees might provide complete financial support for the other functions of the college.

Unfortunately, these noble efforts retarded the realization of such a college still further. A school was one thing, but a new omnipotent licensing board was quite another. One might be willing to give a new school some autonomy, but few were prepared to give it complete dominion over an entire profession. The question of licensing was largely responsible for the endless arguments and delay over the next few years.

After reviewing the proposal, Charles III forwarded it to the Council with instructions to consult Pedro Virgili and Pedro Perchet. The Council immediately complied.[11] Indeed, Charles III habitually sought the advice of renowned individuals before acting. This practice was especially salutary in the case of surgery, for most of the practitioners who had won renown, titles, and government positions were closely

11. Expediente del nuevo Colegio. I have not been able to identify Perchet except for the fact that he, like Virgili, possessed the title *Cirujano de Cámara*.

associated with the progressive surgeons in the College of San Fernando. And most members of the college held government positions or titles, whereas the romance surgeons had none of their own to represent their interests at court.

As might be expected, Virgili and Perchet enthusiastically endorsed the idea of a Madrid school. Such a school, they declared, was "indispensable." They added, however, that the original plan should be adjusted so as to conform with the structure of Barcelona and Cádiz.[12]

By now the idea of a college in Madrid had captured the imagination of Campomanes. He even dreamed of several new colleges to relieve the terrible shortage of Latin surgeons. (The original idea of improving romance surgery seems to have been forgotten.) The Council, though, decided first to consult the Protomedicato and the famous Academy of Medicine.[13] There was heated discussion in both groups. One can imagine one faction insisting that only physicians could be relied upon to maintain standards, while others insisted that a new school could only benefit everyone.

The Academy of Medicine responded first. Although its members recognized the need for surgeons, they assumed that surgery would always be a minor craft and could not understand why an entire school must be devoted to it. In addition, the proposed autonomy from the Protomedicato could be very dangerous. Standards might rapidly decline even further. Moreover, a few schools would have little influence upon surgery as a whole. Would it not be wiser to raise the level of the private instruction already in existence? The academy also had valid objections to the Barcelona school. Most surgical practice concerned simple procedures such as bloodletting, it correctly observed, but the Barcelona professors emphasized newer and bolder operations with which the average surgeon would never come in contact.[14]

Unlike most opponents of San Carlos, the Academy of Medicine was not merely fighting for traditional privileges. Indeed, many of its objections would come to have much validity. The College of San Carlos would never train more than a handful of surgeons, while other instruction probably suffered as most of the government's medical resources were poured into the colleges. And, as is often the case in

12. Dictamen de Pedro Perchet y Pedro Virgili, July 10, 1768, in Consulta sobre cirugía.

13. Repuesta fiscal, Nov. 14, 1768, in Consulta sobre cirugía.

14. Informe de la Real Academia de Medicina de Madrid, Nov. 21, 1768, in Consulta sobre cirugía.

research hospitals even today, San Carlos professors did exhibit much greater interest in the rare diseases and novel procedures than in the more mundane, everyday needs of the sick.

Even so, not all members of the academy agreed. A surgeon, Agustín Navarro, argued that the proposed school was indispensable. Complete separation of medicine and surgery, as existed in France, was highly desirable. The Protomedicato should be forbidden to license surgeons. The school should also be independent of the hospital.[15]

The response of the Protomedicato was far more critical, not only of the proposal but of surgeons in general. Though the physicians praised the emphasis on practical surgery—which romance surgeons already had—they argued that the recommended academic courses would be extremely difficult for surgeons and that classes in the natural sciences would be a complete waste. Why teach a surgeon what he could never use? Let the universities educate anyone who really wanted to become a Latin surgeon.[16]

A year later, in 1770, the fiscal of the Protomedicato, Tomás Toben de Salas, had a change of heart. He wrote a short note to the Council in which he acknowledged the valuable service Barcelona and Cádiz were performing. His only opposition to a school in Madrid, he declared, was its potential autonomy in granting licenses.[17]

Campomanes carefully reviewed the situation and concluded that the legal structure of medicine, particularly the Protomedicato, was at the root of the problem. Surgeons were ignorant and incompetent. Charlatans were everywhere. The countless subdivisions of specialties perpetuated by the Protomedicato created chaos. It was ridiculous to classify practitioners according to the type of treatment they offered. The Protomedicato tried to preserve all faculties for itself, and meanwhile it licensed outright quacks because its members did not know enough surgery to examine candidates in the field. He urged the Council to consider carefully the subordinate role the Protomedicato must observe in public health and the advance of medicine.

Campomanes then turned to the question of a college similar to the one in Barcelona. He vigorously urged the Council to approve the founding of such a school in the Hospital General. A college of surgery in Madrid could create surgeons for the entire kingdom who might replace the romance surgeons and bleeders that now plagued it. It

15. Informe de Agustín Navarro, n.d., in Consulta sobre cirugía.
16. Informe del Protomedicato, n.d., in Consulta sobre cirugía.
17. Informe de Tomás Toben de Salas, n.d., in Consulta sobre cirugía.

should not only be self-governing but empowered to license its own students. To be successful, the school would need an anatomical theater, instruments, and a library. Competent professors were readily available. Campomanes noted that such a school was not a radical innovation; two already existed. The immediate problems were the opposition of the Protomedicato and the lack of funds to finance it.[18]

Thus, the proposals of Campomanes approved not only a college of surgery but a restructuring of the medical profession in which the college would play a vital part. Once again educational reform became a device to reduce the influence of a semiautonomous profession that seemed wedded to the status quo. At the same time, Campomanes's conclusions guaranteed government support for those surgeons intent on transforming their craft into a respected profession.

The Council of Castile formally approved Campomanes's recommendations and forwarded them to the Crown along with background information. In addition, the Council expansively suggested similar schools of surgery in eight other Spanish cities. It was now August 1774. It had been twenty-one years since a Madrid college was first suggested, and six years had passed since Custodio Gutiérrez had submitted the plan that the Council had requested in the first place. One wonders if Campomanes suspected that another thirteen years would pass before this recommendation to his monarch became a reality.

Having been approved in principle by the Council of Castile, the future of a Madrid college of surgery now lay in the hands of Charles III and his personal advisers. After studying the recommendation of the Council he turned to individual surgeons to work out the details. In 1774 he sent Antonio Gimbernat, a professor at Barcelona, and Mariano Rivas, a professor at Cádiz, to study the latest methods of teaching surgery abroad. Gimbernat and Rivas were by no means the first surgeons to study outside Spain, but in this case the two men were not only "to improve themselves in surgery" but also "to bring back observations on [surgical] studies, operations, methods, and the regulations in those nations, schools, and hospitals where training and administration are so much better."[19]

Antonio Gimbernat was one of Spain's most prominent surgeons. He was one of those rare historical figures who possessed the best qualities of intellectual, scholar, politician, administrator, and teacher.

18. Dictamen del Fiscal, Oct. 19, 1771, in Consulta sobre cirugía.

19. The instructions are summarized in AHN, Consejos, Leg. 1368e (Libro de Gobierno), fol. 254–260, Real cédula, April 13, 1780.

Historians of medicine know him for his discovery of the crural arch and his perfection of a method of operating upon it.[20] Luis Sánchez Granjel, the Spanish medical historian, called Gimbernat's discovery the only real anatomical advance of the eighteenth century made by a Spaniard.[21]

Like Pedro Virgili, Antonio Gimbernat was a Catalonian.[22] He was born in a small town in Tarragona in 1734, the son of a notary. After a typical primary education—Latin, grammar, philosophy, and theology—he attended the progressive University of Cervera where he earned a bachelor of arts degree. By this time he had probably heard of Pedro Virgili, a fellow Tarragonan of humble birth who had earned a considerable reputation. Gimbernat, perhaps seeing Virgili as something of an idol, decided to devote his own life to surgery. He applied to the new school of surgery at Cádiz and began his studies there in 1756. Two years later he became an intern, which provided him with greater experience plus a monthly stipend. He spent much of his spare time with the dissector and so impressed the faculty that they appointed him to substitute for the professor of anatomy before Gimbernat even graduated. In 1764 Pedro Virgili appointed him to the chair of anatomy at the new Barcelona school, where he remained until he began his travels in 1774.

In addition to teaching, Gimbernat was constantly searching for new techniques and better procedures. The Barcelona school offered young scientists many opportunities to carry on research and present lectures on their findings. Gimbernat took advantage of these opportunities. In addition to his operation for a crural hernia, which he first performed before his colleagues in 1772, he developed better techniques for operating on the eye and studied the flow of fluids through the liver. He constantly emphasized that one could not perform any surgical technique successfully without thoroughly understanding the anatomy

20. The crural arch (ligamentum inguinale) is a ligament in the lower pelvis. The operation was used to treat hernias. *Dorland's Illustrated Medical Dictionary* (23rd ed.; Philadelphia, 1957), p. 751, also refers to this as "Gimbernat's ligament."

21. Sánchez Granjel, *Anatomía española*, p. 68.

22. Biographical data are from Agustín de Gimbernat, *Sucinta noticia del S.D. Antonio de Gimbernat* (Barcelona, 1828), pp. 14–34 (hereinafter cited as Gimbernat, *Noticia de Gimbernat*. The author was the son of Antonio Gimbernat.); Enrique Salcedo y Ginestal, "Parte biográfica," in Antonio de Gimbernat, *Obras de Don Antonio de Gimbernat precedidas de un estudio biobibliográfico del mismo*, ed. Enrique Salcedo y Ginestal (2 vols.; "Biblioteca Clásica de la Medicina Española," vols. VI–VII; Madrid, 1926–1928), I, 25–212 (hereinafter cited as Salcedo y Ginestal, "Parte biográfica," in *Obras de Gimbernat*.); García del Real, *Historia de la medicina en España*, pp. 449–455; Hernández Morejón, *Historia bibliográfica*, VI, 285–287.

of the region involved. It was his background in anatomy, he later remarked, that led him to discover his new technique for hernias. His principal published work on the crural hernia operation shows him to have been very modern in his research methods.[23] In addition to describing the procedures, the book thoroughly documents several case studies, including their related problems and postoperative recovery. For Gimbernat, surgery was much more than the operation itself. At the same time he eschewed the temptation to explore the philosophical implications of medicine as so many Spanish men of medicine have been accustomed to do. Philosophy, he later wrote, wastes valuable time better devoted to improving one's technical skills.[24]

During his Barcelona years Gimbernat became increasingly concerned about the decadent state of Spanish surgery, the gross ignorance of most practitioners, and the barbarous procedures they used. In the inaugural lecture he delivered in 1768 he looked back to the day when surgeons were "venerated as gods and rewarded with rare privileges." Perhaps, he mused, if the efforts of this school were duplicated throughout Spain, surgery might once again be restored to such a position. Indeed, Gimbernat looked upon himself less as a participant in the growth of modern science than as a crusader fighting for the surgical profession. Surgery, he declared, was among the most important of all the sciences; the ideal surgeon was virtuous, prudent, merciful, imaginative, and intelligent. The historical portion of his address treated surgery as though it had evolved apart from the other sciences. Significantly, he praised Charles III not for his support of science but for his concern for the health of his subjects.[25]

Gimbernat and Rivas[26] studied abroad from 1774 until late in 1778. In Paris they inspected the College of Surgery and worked on the preparations for clinical instruction that the Hôtel Dieu established in 1787. Proceeding to London, they audited the lectures of John Hunter (1728–1793), who more than anyone else was responsible for surgery's becoming a real science. In both his private classes and the public lec-

23. *Nuevo método de operar en la hernia crural* (Madrid, 1793). See pp. 41–42 for the importance of anatomy.

24. Informe, Sept. 6, 1806, quoted in Tomás Carreras y Artau, *Estudios sobre médicos-filósofos españoles del siglo XIX* (Barcelona, 1952), p. 24. Carreras y Artau considers Virgili and Gimbernat very atypical in Spanish medicine for this reason.

25. Antonio Gimbernat, *Oración inaugural, que para la abertura de los estudios celebrada en el Real Colegio de Cirugía de Barcelona* (Barcelona, 1768). The pamphlet is in the library of the Academy of Medicine in Madrid.

26. I have been unable to find biographical material on Rivas. In any event, his contribution was minimal.

tures that attracted students from all over Europe, Hunter stressed the need for a thorough grounding in anatomy. He also developed more intricate techniques of operating and urged surgeons to tie arterial ligatures in healthy tissue above a wound in order to break blood clots. After one lecture Gimbernat approached Hunter and described his technique for the crural hernia operation. Hunter was impressed and added that he would incorporate Gimbernat's discovery into his future lectures.[27] The two Spaniards next went north to Edinburgh, "probably the leading medical center internationally,"[28] and finally to the clinic at Leyden where Boerhaave had taught.

While Gimbernat and Rivas were learning much about the state of surgery in the rest of Europe, Charles III turned to his personal advisers for assistance in solving the more mundane problems of the school at home. Many details still had to be settled, including the touchy question of the relationship between the school and the Protomedicato.

The monarch relied particularly upon his old acquaintance, José Fernández de Miranda, whom he had brought with him when he had returned to Spain in 1759 to assume his crown.[29] Charles gave his close friend the title Duque de Losada and appointed him to the important post of Sumiller de Corps (lord chamberlain). As such, Losada supervised the monarch's personal attendants, including his physicians and surgeons, even though he had had no medical training himself. Losada appointed progressive men to these posts, including graduates of the surgical colleges, and passed on their suggestions for medical reform to Charles himself. Thus, the progressive faction of the medical profession was able to bypass the Protomedicato in their communications with the Crown. Indeed, since 1770, Losada had repeatedly expressed his support of a surgical school in Madrid.[30]

In February 1776 the king sent the entire dossier on the college to

27. Gimbernat proudly relates the whole incident in his *Nuevo método*, pp. 23–24. It obviously meant much to him to have had the approval of a foreign expert with the reputation of Hunter.

28. Ackerknecht, *Medicine at the Paris Hospital*, p. 27.

29. There is little information about Losada. He is mentioned in Antonio Ferrer del Rio, *Historia del reinado de Carlos III en España* (4 vols.; Madrid, 1856), I, 251–252.

30. AGS, Gracia y Justicia, Leg. 405 (900), Copia de expediente sobre la reforma de la cirugía, enviado al Tribunal del Real Protomedicato, Informe de Duque de Losada, May 1, 1776. This expediente, hereinafter cited as Expediente sobre la reforma de la cirugía, contains the correspondence between Losada and the Crown between 1776 and 1779.

his counselor for comments. In response, Losada carefully stressed the importance of making the school independent of the Protomedicato. He agreed in general with the proposals of the Council and suggested that the school might be located in the Botanical Gardens. In addition, he proposed similar schools of pharmacy and chemistry. However, Losada adamantly opposed the idea that the school should license all surgeons. In the first place, he argued, if every school granted licenses, there would be no uniformity among recipients. Moreover, any institution with complete autonomy would be dangerous. The traditional Spanish distinction between the degree and the license to practice was a valuable safeguard. The school should devote all its efforts to education; regulation was a job in itself. Nevertheless, Losada continued, the present superiority of medicine was equally undesirable. As a solution, Losada proposed that the Protomedicato be divided into three separate boards (medicine, surgery, pharmacy), each of which would regulate its proper field. Then graduates of the college would go before a "*Proto-cirujano*" for their license. Medicine would no longer wield power over surgery, but surgery itself would remain under a single governing body.[31]

Losada's comments were sent to the Council, which felt that the Hospital General would be a better location. Aside from the location, the Council agreed with all of Losada's recommendations. Slowly the plans became more concrete as various advisers suggested additional refinements.[32] The Crown sent all the additional reports back to Losada.

In March 1779 Losada presented his final report to the king. The Protomedicato should be divided into three departments as he had previously suggested. A college of surgery for Latin surgeons should be established in the Hospital General, and the Crown should invite Antonio Gimbernat and Mariano Rivas to draw up the ordinances for the new school. Losada added that the ordinances should include a provision whereby professorships would be won through oposición, not by appointment as at Barcelona.[33]

Finally, on May 26, 1779, the Crown issued the long-awaited decree ordering the establishment of a school of surgery in the Hospital Gen-

31. *Ibid.*

32. Expediente del nuevo Colegio summarizes the communications between 1776 and 1779.

33. Informe de Duque de Losada, March 13, 1779, in Expediente sobre la reforma de la cirugía.

eral of Madrid.[34] It would be completely autonomous from the Protomedicato as the College of San Fernando had originally advocated. At the same time the Crown accepted Losada's proposal that a separate board of surgery, not the new college, license practitioners. Thus, the Crown gave the surgeons the school they wanted without entrusting them with the power to govern the profession.

Spanish surgeons no doubt rejoiced that they had finally won freedom from what Custodio Gutiérrez had called "the persecution and tyrannical rule" of the Protomedicato.[35] Surgeons would now license and regulate their fellow surgeons, for the decree carefully divided the Protomedicato into three separate boards to govern the three faculties of medicine, surgery, and pharmacy. Members of all the boards would receive the same salaries and possess identical privileges. Each board was responsible for granting all licenses in its respective science throughout Castile. The Sumiller de Corps was to appoint the proto-cirujanos, one of whom had to be a professor at the Madrid school.

Although there were undoubtedly valid reasons for restricting the physicians, the new tripartite arrangement would be no panacea. Once the school was established, surgeons there would again press their demands for complete licensing powers. In addition, the partition of the Protomedicato ran counter to contemporary trends toward unity. In the eyes of a public long convinced that surgery was inferior to medicine, separation tended to confirm the popular prejudice against the surgeon. Ironically, in later years conservatives fought to maintain the separation while reformers tried to reunite the faculties.

The provisions of the decree regarding the school itself were less controversial. Gimbernat and Rivas were to offer advice on the ordinances for the new school, using the valuable knowledge they had gained abroad. The Crown also endorsed Losada's ideas and instructed the two surgeons to follow them. The First Surgeon of His Majesty was to be president of the college. Professors were to win their positions through oposición and were to receive a higher salary than their counterparts in Barcelona because Madrid had a higher cost of living.

34. Real orden, May 26, 1779, in Expediente sobre la reforma de la cirugía. Another copy is in AGS, Gracia y Justicia, Leg. 404 (989). An almost identical Real cédula was issued on April 13, 1780, after Gimbernat had been consulted. This cédula is in AHN, Consejos, Leg. 1368e (Libro de Gobierno), fol. 254–260, and is summarized in *Nov. Rec.* VIII, xii, 1.

35. AGS, Gracia y Justicia, Leg. 404 (989), Representación de Pedro Custodio Gutiérrez, n.d.

Students were to be encouraged to practice their art in rural villages after graduation.

By 1779 Pedro Custodio Gutiérrez, the architect of the original 1768 plan, was First Surgeon of the king and destined to become president of the Madrid school. Perhaps he was irritated at the changes made in his original proposal. At any rate, he wrote copious notes in the margin of a copy of the 1779 order in which he criticized the dissimilarity between the Madrid school and the one in Barcelona.[36] (One could make the same criticism of his own original proposal.) It was ridiculous to encourage students from all of Spain to apply to the school since it would never be able to accommodate them. He reiterated his plea for the school itself to grant licenses. Professors would otherwise be restricted in their teaching by the need to cater to examinations, and the school would be deprived of a valuable source of revenue. Moreover, the First Surgeon complained, the task of drawing up a curriculum had been relegated to two surgeons "who cannot be considered as thoroughly educated as some others."

The criticisms were ignored. In April 1780 Gimbernat and Rivas took up residence in the Hospital General and began work on the ordinances, guided by the criteria set out in the royal order of the preceding year.[37] Over the next few years the two men submitted several reports on their progress to the Council and to Losada.

In July Gimbernat offered the Crown a general picture of the school he had in mind, an eclectic synthesis of the best he had seen in Europe.[38] It would have a large amphitheater seating four hundred persons for anatomical dissections. Connected to the theater would be a smaller room where students could practice dissections themselves. There would be a library, a classroom, a room for keeping instruments, and a collection of "natural and artificial" anatomical pieces to demonstrate various disorders and operative methods. All the rooms would be bright and well ventilated. The staff would include a director, eight professors, a secretary, and a librarian who could read French, Italian, and English. In sum, he concluded, the school would have the same facilities as the best schools in France, England, Scotland, and Holland, and he hoped the Madrid school would carry on correspondence with the schools in those countries.

36. The notes are on the copy in AGS, Gracia y Justicia, Leg. 404 (989).

37. "Oficio a los Sres. Gimbernat y Rivas," April 8, 1780, in *Obras de Gimbernat*, II, 135–143.

38. "Informe sobre el establecimiento del Colegio de Cirugía de Madrid dado por D. Antonio Gimbernat," July 14, 1780, in *Obras de Gimbernat*, II, 145–154.

Most eighteenth-century medical reformers realized the importance of anatomy, but Gimbernat believed that practical experience was equally essential. "Surgery is a practical skill; it must be learned not only through study and hearing explanations, but also by working and observing . . . the patient." To provide this practical experience Gimbernat proposed a clinic for some fifty patients. About twenty students would reside at the school to assist in their care. Finally, Gimbernat observed that obstetrics, which was considered an essential part of surgery abroad, should be included in the curriculum.

By the end of 1781 Gimbernat decided not simply to duplicate the curriculum at Barcelona.[39] This would only perpetuate its shortcomings. The new school would have eight professors instead of five and offer instruction in eye diseases, obstetrics, and the basic facts of internal diseases that were so often at the root of surgical problems. A five-year course would rationally instill in the student a thorough understanding of surgery: anatomy to teach the structure of the body, physiology to show it in operation, the science of hygiene to describe the body in a state of health, pathology to study the unhealthy body, and therapeutics to teach how to cure the unhealthy body. In addition, the student would study operations, *materia medica*, and those diseases that require surgical procedures but have internal causes (*afectos mixtos*). This precise order of courses was essential, Gimbernat explained, for a student had to be familiar with the body in a state of health before he could understand disease. He suggested up-to-date texts for the courses–Boerhaave, Winslow, and others–but relied upon the professor to synthesize the material for his course. Thus, every course would be based on content, not on authors.

Gimbernat was equally specific on the requirements for matriculation. These requirements had to be strict as one of the objectives of the school was to improve the unfavorable popular view of surgery. Applicants would have to be proficient in Latin, logic, algebra and geometry, and physics. Moreover, they would have to prove their limpieza de sangre by submitting proof of the baptism and good life and habits of themselves, their parents, and their grandparents. Gimbernat made it clear, however, that he was imposing these strict standards of ancestry in order to assure the good name of the school and the profession. "If candidates for a license in surgery are prepared with

39. "Informe para el régimen y gobierno del Real Colegio de Cirugía de Madrid dado por D. Antonio de Gimbernat y D. Mariano Ribas," Dec. 31, 1781, in *Obras de Gimbernat*, II, 155–198.

no other test than their studies, there will always be some who, by virtue of their ancestry or conduct, will preserve surgery in the decadent state it is." In other words, Gimbernat was determined that future surgeons would not harm the good name of the profession. One's family background was important in the eighteenth century. Whether Gimbernat personally felt that limpieza de sangre was important in judging a man is unclear, but it is certain that public opinion put great stock in such things. For similar reasons he also proposed prohibiting students from accepting part-time jobs as barbers' assistants. He feared any association of the school with barbers would harm its good name.

The formal structure of the college promised to make it unique. Although advanced surgical training existed in many places, and France possessed colleges of surgery, Gimbernat's regulations imposed requirements for matriculation and graduation that existed nowhere else. Thus, to the extent that the transformation of surgery was related to the establishment of profession-like standards, Spanish surgeons would be considerably ahead of their colleagues elsewhere.

In the meantime Gimbernat had been appointed an examiner of surgery in the reorganized Protomedicato. He and his fellow examiners were shocked at the applicants who came before them. Most were completely ignorant; some could barely read. They had memorized a few facts and hoped to pass the exam by reciting them back. Gimbernat believed incompetent teachers were largely responsible. Accordingly, the board petitioned the Council for permission to certify which master surgeons would be allowed to accept students, and to permit only their students to take the examination. Approved teachers were to hold regular classes in which they taught some anatomy, physiology, and pathology. Campomanes doubted that a sufficient number of qualified teachers could be found, but he agreed to the request, as did the Council. Eleven surgeons applied for the certification. Most of the five accepted later taught at San Carlos. The Council, meanwhile, was immediately inundated with requests for it to make exceptions. The whole affair was but an interim effort until the college opened. It was not very effective—the exceptions appear to have been granted readily—but it had given Gimbernat another opportunity to impress on the Council the urgency of the situation.[40]

40. AHN, Consejos, Leg. 924, Exp. 22, Parte 1, Expediente . . . sobre nombramiento de profesores, 1780–1783. This contains the *informes* of Gimbernat et al., Nov. 22, 1780, and Oct. 31, 1782; the *dictámenes* of the fiscal; and *representaciones* of various surgeons.

Between 1780 and 1787 countless memos and reports passed among the two surgeons, the Duque de Losada, and the Council of Castile. Meanwhile, the Protomedicato and the Royal Board of Hospitals (*Real Junta de Hospitales*) continued to oppose the new school and its promised autonomy.[41] The location also remained a problem. Gimbernat suggested a new building connected to the Hospital de la Pasión, the more modern women's hospital near the Hospital General. The Crown ordered construction started there in 1783, but this work never reached completion until the 1830s. For a while the situation looked desperate since the animosity of the Board of Hospitals made the Hospital General undesirable as a site. In 1786 Gimbernat had to suggest renting a private dwelling as a temporary measure. Fortunately, however, his diplomatic talents finally enabled him to win over the Board of Hospitals. As a result the basement of the new addition at the Hospital General was set aside for his temporary use.[42]

Financial support for the school proved to be less of a problem. In 1783 the Crown promised the school an annual subsidy of 18,000 *reales de vellón*, which would start in 1786.[43] This was a substantial sum, considering that it did not include salaries, which were appropriated separately. The Crown also began compensating Gimbernat and Rivas with 30,000 reales annually and provided funds for two of the future professors to study in Paris and London. Three years later the remaining officers of the school began receiving their salaries according to a scale drawn up by Gimbernat.[44] The Crown's generous financial support of the school not only helped guarantee its success but also assured its complete independence from the Protomedicato and the Board of Hospitals.

41. According to the Marqués de Valdecarzana, who succeeded Losada as *Sumiller de Corps* and was similarly sympathetic toward the college, the physicians on the Protomedicato did their best to make it all but impossible for Gimbernat and his fellow surgeons to function effectively. (AGS, Gracia y Justicia, Leg. 405 [991], Informe del Marqués de Valdecarzana, April 11, 1785.)

42. Expediente del nuevo Colegio contains the details of this correspondence. See also Salcedo de Ginestal, "Parte biográfica," in *Obras de Gimbernat*, I, 218–222.

43. This *Real resolución*, which I was unable to locate, is described in AHN, Consejos, Leg. 1035, Exp. 1, Parte 1, *Real Cédula de S.M. y Señores del Consejo, en que se aprueban y mandan observar las Ordenanzas formadas para el Gobierno económico y escolástico del Colegio de Cirugía, establecido en Madrid con el título de San Carlos* (Madrid, 1787), Feb. 24, 1787. (The cédula is hereinafter cited as *Cédula del Colegio de San Carlos.*)

44. For details on pre-1787 finances, see Archivo de la Facultad de Medicina de la Universidad de Madrid (hereinafter AFM), Libro de Representaciones, Ordenes y Repuestas, y Reales Cédulas, 1787–1817 (hereinafter cited as Libro de Representaciones, Ordenes, etc.), Informe del Colegio, April 8, 1790. This Libro contains the full text of all such documents.

Now that final approval of the ordinances seemed imminent, final preparations began for the opening of the school. The 1786 government subsidy went to purchase articles for teaching anatomy, the first course students would take. These items included two volumes of engravings by Gautier,[45] wax and plaster models, and various utensils to enable the school to make additional models of its own. Ignacio Lacaba, the future dissector of the college, immediately set to work preparing exhibits. That July he placed on display a heart, a skeleton, a model of a head, and one of an entire body. Gimbernat contributed some additional pieces from his own collection. Meanwhile, there were more mundane items to acquire—cabinets, desks, carpets, and paper. But Gimbernat was thrifty; at the end of the year 15,000 reales remained in the treasury.[46]

Finally, on February 24, 1787, the Crown approved the ordinances for the school, dubbed it San Carlos, and ordered it to open the following October. The statutes, in the main, followed the earlier recommendations of Gimbernat. The president of the college would be His Majesty's First Surgeon. A director would supervise its day-to-day operation. He and eight professors would make up a governing junta. The statutes thoroughly described the content and rationale of each course, the practical exercises, the clinic, the anatomical dissections, the resident students, and the requirements for matriculation and graduation. The section on government, finances, and the duties of various officers seemed to provide for every contingency.[47]

The ordinances generally followed those of Barcelona. Like its predecessor, San Carlos would provide its students with a thorough grounding in anatomy and the opportunity to practice operative techniques on cadavers. The new statutes, however, included the innovations Gimbernat had proposed. They provided for daily experience in

45. Gautier d'Agoty (1717–1786) was a French engraver who had no medical training himself. Garrison, *An Introduction to the History of Medicine*, p. 335, describes his work as very artistic but too gaudy for classroom use.

46. AFM, Libro de Cuentas: Entradas y Salidas del Caudal de Dotación Señalado al Real Colegio de San Carlos, 1786–1815 (hereinafter cited as Libro de Cuentas [1786–1815]). For Gimbernat's interest and contributions, see Salcedo y Ginestal, "Parte biográfica," in *Obras de Gimbernat*, I, 237–238. For details on the collection, see *Memorial Literario Instructivo y Curioso de la Corte de Madrid*, July, 1786, pp. 373 ff.

47. *Ordenanzas del Real Colegio de Cirugía en Madrid con el título de San Carlos* (Madrid, 1787). The printed ordinances, hereinafter cited as *Ordenanzas* (1787), are part of the *Cédula del Colegio de San Carlos*. Copies of the ordenanzas exist in AHN, Consejos, Leg. 1035, Exp. 1, Parte 1, and ADP, Leg. 118. The statutes themselves will be more thoroughly discussed in the following chapters.

a clinic. Therapeutics and pathology, one of the youngest but most promising branches of medicine, received greater attention. Students would acquire at least a rudimentary knowledge of internal medicine, pharmacology, and obstetrics.

These refinements, which came at an important juncture in the history of medicine, further testify to the farsightedness of Antonio Gimbernat. Spanish surgeons had been grossly ignorant of basic anatomy, and the earlier schools and universities were right to call for its restoration. By the late eighteenth century, however, ignorance of human anatomy was no longer the principal barrier to more advanced surgical procedures. Until anesthetics and the need for sterilization were known, the surgeon was circumscribed in what he could accomplish no matter how sophisticated his knowledge of bones and muscles. The new frontiers of medical science lay in physiology and pathology, especially morbid pathology. From these younger sciences nineteenth-century medicine would score important achievements in understanding the nature of disease. Thus, the graduates of San Carlos would be better prepared than most to cope with the future developments of their discipline.

In the cédula that accompanied the publication of the ordinances, the Crown named Gimbernat and Rivas co-directors in perpetuity and granted them a lifetime pension of 12,000 reales in addition to their salaries. Gimbernat would go on to become First Surgeon of His Majesty, and Rivas later received an appointment at the Royal Palace at Aranjuez.[48] Assuredly both men deserved their rewards for their diligent efforts.

Although the statutes followed Losada's suggestion and required an oposición for all chairs, the Crown decided to appoint the original professors of the school. Presumably Gimbernat had recommended them. The members of that first illustrious faculty represented the aristocracy of Spanish surgery: a professor each from Barcelona and Cádiz, a surgeon of the Royal Guards, a professor at the Royal Studies of San Isidro, a member of the Royal Medical Society of Seville, two surgeons-major in the army, and, of course, Gimbernat and Rivas.[49] All were Latin surgeons, closely in touch with the most recent progress in their discipline; all held well-paid, highly respected positions. This faculty alone promised that education at San Carlos would rank among the best in Europe.

48. On Rivas, see ARP, Sección de Empleados, Exp. de Mariano Rivas.
49. *Cédula del Colegio de San Carlos.*

Thus, after more than three decades, a college of surgery in Madrid was finally a reality. The events of the intervening years reveal much about the relationship between reformers and the government, the importance of regulatory powers, and the character of the progressive surgeons themselves.

The school itself was the creation of surgeons, from its initial conception to the details of its day-to-day operation. The Council only received their suggestions, studied them, and commissioned others to work out the details so that they might be put into effect. Yet it was the receptiveness of the Council to such proposals in the first place that prevented them from becoming lost in some government file.

The Council consistently acted with extreme caution. It reached no decision without carefully reviewing the opinions of all concerned. Its zealous efforts to avoid acting capriciously led to long delays. Even Charles himself hesitated to act on the recommendations of his Council without consulting his personal adviser, the Duque de Losada. It was primarily the controversy over regulation and licensing, not the school itself, that led to the interminable delays. Certainly the debate itself illustrates the complete scorn and lack of respect physicians and surgeons felt for each other. Progressive surgeons, in particular, had no confidence in the established medical profession. One can detect their anger and frustration at being treated like mere tradesmen by the very Protomedicato that had allowed incompetent surgeons to practice in the first place. If surgery were ever to become a respected profession, it must be governed by surgeons.

The Council and the Duque de Losada sympathized with these frustrations and agreed that the Protomedicato had failed to regulate surgery adequately. At the same time, however, they saw the wisdom in the traditional distinction between education and licensing, and were determined to avoid creating a new autonomous body that was contradictory to their policy of centralization, national standards, and royal control. The compromise worked out by Losada solved the dilemma.

To be sure, the surgeons who created San Carlos were unrepresentative of their profession, and the school reflected this. Most surgeons were of the working class, but the small group associated with the college held royal titles, received high salaries, and lived with the elite of Spanish society. Indeed, many of this reformist element had been raised in a poor, rural environment, but their education had taken them from it. Although this "class distinction" within the profession can easily be overemphasized, it seems clear that the reformist surgeon did consider himself a cut above the ordinary. He saw himself as a professional and intellectual, and wanted the medical profession to accept him as such.

Perhaps the ambiguous position of the educated Spanish surgeon led to his preoccupation with foreign models. The advocates of reform constantly pointed to England, Scotland, and Holland to buttress their arguments. Gimbernat carefully constructed his school to resemble what he had seen outside Spain. To be sure, he was very selective in choosing his foreign models; Spain would imitate only the best. Nevertheless, Spanish surgical reformers, though always themselves Spaniards, were ever conscious of the latest in medical education elsewhere.

The ambitions and frustrations of the progressive educated surgeons may also have led to the creation of the college that was not designed to increase the number of practicing surgeons as rapidly as possible. The professors of the College of San Fernando who had originally proposed a school of surgery were primarily concerned about the incompetence of the average practicing romance surgeon. The College of San Carlos, however, ignored the mass of practicing surgeons and chose to train a small number of real scientists instead. In a sense, the founders of San Carlos hoped for perfection for a few rather than improvement for many. The curricula seemed designed more for the potential research scholar than for the average practitioner; indeed, the entrance requirements made it impossible for most romance surgeons to matriculate.

During the months following the publication of the ordinances, the new staff worked on the final preparations. The governing junta began holding weekly meetings every Thursday. It immediately purchased additional wax figures of parts of the body and bought the necessary instruments for performing dissections from craftsmen in Madrid and Barcelona. Some of the professors busied themselves preparing a list of books for the library. The Crown forwarded the book list to Paris and London so that the Spanish ambassadors there might buy them.[50] By autumn the new school already had a reputation abroad. The director of the Royal Academy of Surgery in Paris wrote offering to send the school all of its publications in return for those of San

50. AFM, Libro de Representaciones, Ordenes, etc., Real orden, June 21, 1787, and Aviso, July 20, 1787.

Carlos.[51] The connections Gimbernat had made abroad would serve the school well.

One unforeseen problem arose, however, that would continue to plague the school in the future. This was a serious lack of qualified students. Apparently few educated young men were ready to embark on a career in surgery. Publicity for the new institution began back in early May with an announcement in the official *Gaceta de Madrid.* It contained a glowing description of the college and invited prospective students to apply. It also listed entrance requirements: three years of Latin and logic, and one year each of algebra, geometry, and experimental physics.[52] By the end of September, only three applicants had met the qualifications. After serious discussion, the college junta decided that the algebra, geometry, and physics were the stumbling block since relatively few schools taught these subjects. Accordingly, the junta petitioned the Crown to suspend the science requirements for three years. It hoped that by that time prospective students would be better aware of the requirements and that secondary education would have improved. The Crown eventually agreed in February 1788. But it was too late. Only three students attended San Carlos during its inaugural year, and only a single new one matriculated the following year.[53]

At any rate, the College of San Carlos commenced classes in the art and science of surgery on October 2, 1787. Several auditors helped make the scarcity of students a little less disturbing. The professors gave learned lectures from time to time in formal actos. The library and the collection of anatomical exhibits grew steadily. Members of the Council of Castile attended the second formal opening of classes in October 1788. Gimbernat led the academic procession into the theater. Mariano Rivas gave the oration. It was entitled "The Necessity and Value of Education."[54]

51. AFM, Libro de Acuerdos (1787–1804), Junta of Nov. 13, 1787. The Libros de Acuerdos are basically the minutes of the meetings of the governing junta. The notations primarily consist of summaries of resolutions passed and orders received from superior bodies.

52. *Gaceta de Madrid*, May 4, 1787, pp. 295–296. Documentation of limpieza de sangre was also required.

53. AFM, Libro de Acuerdos (1787–1804), Juntas of Sept. 13, 1787, and Feb. 12, 1788; Libro de Representaciones, Ordenes, etc., Representación de Gimbernat, Oct. 5, 1787; AHN, Consejos, Leg. 3514, Exp. 17, Parte 4, Representación del Colegio de San Carlos, Sept. 23, 1788.

54. AHN, Consejos, Leg. 3514, Exp. 17, Parte 4, Informe de Pablo Ferrándiz Benedicho, n.d. (early Oct. 1788).

CHAPTER V

# ACADEMIC LIFE AND ORGANIZATION AT SAN CARLOS

THE YEARS BETWEEN the opening of San Carlos in 1787 and the French invasion of Spain in 1808 were productive ones for the new college. The education it offered its students was without doubt the equal of any in Europe. The modern authors, the clinical training, and the emphasis on practical experience stood in sharp contrast to the decadent medical training that earlier Spanish writers had criticized. The learned papers and thoughtful criticisms by the school's professors extended the influence of the school still further.

Although San Carlos was intimately involved in the continuing efforts to reform the medical profession as a whole, its principal contributions to eighteenth-century Spanish surgery were academic. Its modern curriculum, which served as a model for reform elsewhere, guaranteed that its graduates would be familiar with the latest medical knowledge. In addition, San Carlos offered a national forum in which new research and techniques could be evaluated and publicized. It provided the profession with public lectures and demonstrations, scholarly criticisms of new discoveries, and a review of new medical literature.

Like most Spanish institutions, San Carlos was governed by lengthy statutes that described every aspect of its operation in meticulous detail. The 1787 ordinance ran to more than one hundred pages. The section on curriculum specified everything—from which books the professor was to use in his lectures to the precise hour and length of each class. Neither professor nor administrator had much opportunity to use his own initiative. One of the major tasks of administration was the frequent petitioning of higher authorities to make the inevitable exceptions to the rule. Approval from higher authority was required even for such minor matters as giving a student credit for a course in which he had missed several classes.[1]

1. Archivo de la Universidad Central, Madrid (hereinafter cited as AUC), Libro

Had the statutes remained the same, their exacting detail would not have been a serious problem; but they did not. The reign of Charles IV (1788–1808) was one of endless tinkering with the institutions of government. The rapid rise and fall of the king's ministers, the French Revolution, and, above all, the impulsiveness of Manuel de Godoy, the real ruler of Spain, all contributed to a state of flux. The ministers of Charles III had acted carefully and deliberately; years of discussion had preceded any serious reform. During the reign of Charles IV, however, radical innovations seemed to occur overnight. To be sure, Godoy considered himself a creature of the Enlightenment. Many of his reforms would have been good ones had the groundwork been more carefully laid and had he not backed down in the face of criticism. As it was, the harm caused by instability and constant change could outweigh any good the reforms might bring about.[2]

This constant tinkering affected San Carlos. In 1795, and again in 1804, the Crown imposed new statutes on the school in an attempt to bring all the surgical colleges into greater conformity. Most of the changes, however, were administrative. The curriculum, the hallmark of Gimbernat's efforts to improve surgery, remained loyal to his principles.

Education at San Carlos stands in stark contrast to that of the universities at the beginning of the eighteenth century; it is fitting testimony to Gimbernat's genius and to the remarkable progress that had occurred in Spanish medicine in only a few generations.[3] The principal achievements of the medical reformers at Salamanca had been to turn to modern authors, to base courses on subject matter rather than authors, and, in a general way, to establish a rational progression of material through the four-year program. Antonio Gimbernat went much further; he accepted the general division of theory and practice, and established four chairs of each. Each chair was devoted to a specific field of knowledge. Presumably, every instructor would teach the

---

de Acuerdos (1804–1810), contains many examples.

The Archivo de la Universidad Central, an uncatalogued, semiprivate collection in an old Ministry of Education building, contains innumerable records of the various institutions that were incorporated into the Central University of Madrid in the 1840s. The College of San Carlos, most of whose records are here, became the faculty of medicine of the university in 1845. In 1967 preparations were under way to transfer the collections to the proper libraries of the University of Madrid.

2. The specific reforms of the legal structure of medicine and medical education, and the corresponding efforts to standardize all medical education, will be examined in the following chapter.

3. The description of the curriculum that follows is primarily based on the ordenanzas of 1787 and 1795. Significant modifications will be noted later.

subject in which he was most expert. In the 1787 plan the theoretical chairs were those in anatomy, physiology and hygiene, pathology and therapeutics, and materia medica. The chairs of practical studies included those of surgical diseases (*afectos quiruricos*), obstetrics and venereal disease, operations, and "mixed diseases" (*afectos mixtos*, i.e., diseases with internal and external symptoms). In 1795 obstetrics and venereal diseases were relegated to separate chairs, and the chair of afectos mixtos became that of medical theory and practice. Gimbernat's description of the curriculum emphasized that the rational progression from one course to the next was as important as the list of courses itself. All classes were interdependent.

Gimbernat not only chose the most up-to-date texts but gave the individual professor considerable leeway in organizing his course. The statutes made it clear that the prescribed authors were to serve only as a guide. The student was to learn the content of the particular discipline, not the totality of one expert's writings. The professor was responsible for being aware of the new books in his specialty and was free to use another text if he chose. Gimbernat expected his teachers to write their lectures rather than plow through a single book. Such a liberal policy was rare in the eighteenth century, but it worked well. In 1794 Gimbernat could justifiably boast that "every professor had done his best to deliver lectures full of the valuable ideas and recent knowledge that he had acquired in his reading, travels, reflection, and observation."[4] Indeed, professors had plenty of time for study and reflection, for they had to spend only one hour a day teaching. Some even had several months or a whole semester without classroom duties.

Gimbernat's concern for the education of future surgeons began with the training they would receive before coming to San Carlos. The 1787 statutes attempted to guarantee that every student would have had a thorough background in mathematics and the natural sciences, but the backward state of most secondary education made this difficult. Every applicant was required to have studied geometry and experimental, or modern, physics. Since they were to become Latin surgeons, they also had to have studied Latin and logic. The sciences would replace the years of philosophy formerly required for a license in Latin surgery. After 1795 prospective students who lacked the physics prerequisite could attend the class at the Royal School of San Isidro during their first year at San Carlos.

4. AFM, Libro de Representaciones, Ordenes, etc., Informe del Colegio de San Carlos, Dec. 6, 1794. As usual, the directors of the college signed the informe.

Although the individual teacher had considerable freedom in his own class, the five-year curriculum as a whole was rigidly fixed. There were no electives. Classes met for sixty minutes every day. There were two semesters, October through February and March through July, although some classes ran only a few months. All classes were conducted in Spanish. As in the universities, students were obliged to attend most courses for two consecutive years. The value of this requirement seems dubious since the student simply heard the same material again, though probably the review was beneficial. At any rate, Gimbernat was definitely pleased with his handiwork. His 1795 statutes, which for the most part repeat those of 1787, describe the plan of studies as "the most perfect education up to now inside and outside Spain."

The new student at San Carlos began his academic career with the study of anatomy, the long-neglected but essential subject that had been the focal point of all medical reformers for so long. Gimbernat, a strong believer in its value and necessity, made sure that it would receive its proper emphasis at San Carlos. So, too, did the other professors. In 1795 Ignacio Lacaba, the anatomy professor, requested and was granted permission to extend the course another month so that he might give "complete instruction."[5]

The instructor first discussed the bone structure of the body, particularly essential for an eighteenth-century surgeon. He then moved on to the various tissues, glands, internal organs, and muscles (sarcology), and concluded the course by describing the "organs of sense." In 1787 Gimbernat chose the *Exposición anotómica* of Jacob Winslow (1669–1760). This systematic work was the standard medical text throughout the eighteenth century. One medical historian has dubbed it "the best all-round treatise on the subject before the nineteenth century."[6] But Gimbernat was not content merely to rely on one good text. His ordinances urged the professor of anatomy to watch for a better source and use it if one were found. Above all, he added, the professor was to keep himself informed of any new discoveries.

5. AFM, Libro de Acuerdos que se remitan a la Junta Superior para su aprobación antes de sentarlos en el libro, 1795–1800 (hereinafter cited as AFM, Libro de Acuerdos para la Junta Superior), Representación del Colegio de San Carlos, Nov. 17, 1795, and Orden de la Junta Superior, Dec. 21, 1795.

The books containing the records of the weekly meetings of the San Carlos junta are variously called Libros de Asuntos and Libros de Acuerdos. The books for the years 1787–1804 are in the AFM; all others are in the AUC. The book cited above, however, contains the exact texts of communications between the college and the Superior Board and is not to be confused with the collections of junta minutes.

6. Garrison, *An Introduction to the History of Medicine*, p. 332. Winslow was also used in the universities after their reform.

The eminent surgeons of San Carlos, in their efforts to raise the intellectual level of Spanish surgery and to encourage domestic research, consistently strove to adopt the writings of Spaniards whenever possible. In 1795 Juan de Dios López, a Spanish author who closely followed Winslow, replaced the Dutch authority. And the following year the college began using the first treatise by one of its own professors. This was the five-volume *Curso completo de anatomía del cuerpo humano* by Jaime Bonells and Ignacio Lacaba (Madrid, 1796), professors of anatomy at Cádiz and San Carlos, respectively. It, too, was similar in content to Winslow's work but superior in its clarity of expression and value as a pedagogical tool.[7]

Like so many of their contemporary reformers, Bonells and Lacaba saw themselves as crusaders striving to eliminate a heritage of ignorance and superstition. They hoped that by making anatomy available to all prospective doctors Spanish medicine would return to its former glory. To be sure, even a nonprofessional examination of their work provides further evidence of the familiarity some Spanish physicians and surgeons now had with the latest advances in their science. They carefully synthesized the discoveries of the greatest scholars of the century —John Hunter, Albrecht von Haller, Paolo Masagni, Pierre-Joseph Desault—thereby improving upon Winslow's work.[8] The text itself was strictly descriptive as befits a classroom aid, and it left aside physiological notions. It thoroughly and logically discussed the bones, muscles, blood vessels, nerves, and major organs, classifying each by composition and location. At last Spanish educators had a book designed specifically for easy learning. It concluded with a practical handbook on performing dissections, conserving the specimens, and even detailed lessons on performing Caesarean sections on deceased women, post-mortem examinations, and embalming.

7. García del Real, *Historia de la medicina en España*, pp. 476–477. A copy of the *Curso completo* is in the library of the Academia de Medicina of Madrid.

Jaime Bonells, from Barcelona, was a physician and author of other more technical works. He was a member of the academies of medicine in Madrid and Paris, and had studied extensively abroad.

Ignacio Lacaba, also from Barcelona, studied surgery at Cádiz and later taught there. In 1787 he became anatomical dissector at San Carlos, where he built up an impressive collection of exhibits. He moved to the chair of anatomy in 1795 and became a member of the Junta Superior de Cirugía in 1804.

8. Bonells and Lacaba, *Curso completo*, I. xxxii–xxxv. For Hunter, see Chap. IV. Albrecht von Haller (1708–1777) wrote a widely used textbook on physiology. Paola Mascagni (1752–1815) was a superb illustrator noted for his accurate detail. Pierre-Joseph Desault (1744–1795) investigated blood vessels.

Learning anatomy, however, entailed far more than attending lectures. In addition to the chair of anatomy, the college had an anatomical dissector to illustrate lectures and assist the students. Most lectures were accompanied by exhibits prepared by the dissector. Moreover, the students were to perform the procedures they had seen in class themselves. A special room (*sala práctica*) was set aside in which students practiced performing dissections and operations. Very rarely did a university student have the opportunity to gain such practical experience under the watchful eye of an expert. The dissector was also responsible for maintaining strict "obedience, respect, and decorum" in the sala práctica at all times. Apparently adolescent exuberance in such awesome surroundings sometimes became excessive. On one occasion the governing junta was forced to have the skeletons placed under lock and key in order to prevent the students from mutilating and breaking them.[9]

The importance of anatomy was further underlined by the requirement that all students attend the class again during their second year. Moreover, much of the limited space in the basement of the Hospital General was given over to that discipline. There was a large hall for public demonstrations, the practice room, and the small museum. What with its constant expenses for transporting cadavers and purchasing instruments and exhibits, instruction in anatomy was also expensive. During its early years the college spent an average of three thousand reales, or one-sixth of its annual subsidy, for such things.[10]

In light of the popular eighteenth-century attitude toward dissection of the human body, it is remarkable that San Carlos apparently had no difficulty in obtaining a sufficient number of cadavers. Although occasionally strained relations with the Hospital General created minor problems, there is no mention in the school's records of a shortage of cadavers at any time. Indeed, attending public anatomical demonstrations seems to have been something of a fashionable pastime for the cultured of Madrid. The ordinances required that the demonstrations be open to the public, and they were well attended. Outsiders began to audit courses at San Carlos, particularly anatomy, as soon as the school opened. Some were prospective students, while others simply had an interest in medicine. In 1795 Ignacio Lacaba requested and received permission to hold the class at six in the afternoon instead of

9. AFM, Libro de Acuerdos (1787–1804), Junta of Oct. 6, 1803.
10. AFM, Libro de Cuentas (1786–1815).

during the mornings so that more "aficionados" might attend.[11] Two years later the limited facilities were insufficient to accommodate everyone who wanted to observe the demonstrations. By 1806 the situation was critical. Diego Rodríquez del Piño, the professor of anatomy, complained that more than two hundred persons were crowding into the small room, creating an unhealthy situation. Moreover, Rodríquez continued, between the closely packed crowd and the odor of the cadaver the air became so stale that he always had a painful headache by the time the class was over. As a temporary solution the partition between the amphitheater and a small office was removed. A few weeks later the classes moved into the larger auditorium of the Hospital General.[12]

Wax figures formed another important part of anatomical instruction in the eighteenth century, both in the classroom and in public displays. Artists competed to render their work as accurate as possible; special collections were displayed in one European capital after another. The English surgeon, John Hunter, built up a collection of some thirteen hundred pieces. Gimbernat was apparently impressed by Hunter's collection, for he suggested one in his first proposals for the school in 1780. From the beginning, the college devoted much attention to building up its own collection. Special craftsmen were essential. In early 1788 a Juan Chávez received a temporary commission to make wax pieces under Gimbernat's supervision. Two years later Luis Francheschi was permanently employed to fashion wax models under the direction of Ignacio Lacaba, with a salary of 6,600 reales a year. By 1797 he had completed a collection on obstetrics and was preparing to begin work on a skeleton showing the major organs and ligaments. Nine years later he turned to models displaying the nervous system. The exhibit continued to receive attention. In 1806 the Crown named two apprentices to assist Francheschi, to learn his craft, and eventually to move into his position.[13]

11. AFM, Libro de Representaciones, Ordenes, etc., Representación del Colegio de San Carlos, Dec. 31, 1795. Also Informes del Colegio de San Carlos, Feb. 21, 1789, Dec. 6, 1794.

12. AUC, Libro de Acuerdos (1804–1810), Juntas of Nov. 13, Nov. 23, 1806. The popularity of the demonstrations is also discussed in Salcedo de Ginestal, "Parte biográfica," *Obras de Gimbernat*, I, 260.

Diego Rodríguez del Piño, a Barcelona native, studied at Cádiz and held the chair of anatomy there before coming to San Carlos in 1799. He was vice-director of San Carlos from 1800 until the chaos of 1809.

13. AFM, Libro de Acuerdos (1787–1804), Junta of March 26, 1788; Libro de Representaciones, Ordenes, etc., Informes del Colegio de San Carlos, Feb. 21, 1789, Dec. 6,

Anatomy, however, was only the first step in the education of future surgeons. Once the student had become familiar with the organs of the body and "their number, shape, location, and size," he proceeded to learn "their functions, movements, and changes."[14] This was the science of physiology and hygiene, and was a sharp break from the traditional training of an apprentice, who most likely came in contact only with patients in need of help.

The course in physiology went from March through July. Students attended the lectures again in the spring of their second year. The professor drew his lectures from the writings of Hermann Boerhaave, Albrecht von Haller, and other contemporaries, although the final course itself was his own. These sources were excellent; Boerhaave's *Institutes* was particularly thorough and well documented in its treatment of physiology. And Haller's *Elementa Physiologiae* (1759–1766) contained all the newer findings of the eighteenth century. Haller was also influential in turning physiology away from speculation to step-by-step investigation, and he was the first to illustrate the distinction between the response to stimuli of nerves and muscles.[15] The San Carlos professor followed Haller's example of illustrating his lectures with experiments.

Finally, during June and July, the first-year student attended classes on bandages (*vendages*) given by the professor of surgical diseases. (The 1795 statutes inexplicably transferred the course to the professor of venereal disease.) The instructor illustrated the methods of applying various types of dressings and bandages on life-size mannequins, and the students then applied the techniques themselves. Treating wounds and applying dressings and bandages was an important part of the surgeon's craft. After a year of difficult theoretical work the student was probably pleased to get down to something concrete. Second-year students repeated the course.

Much of the second year at San Carlos was a repetition of the first, with more experience in the anatomical sala de práctica. By the second semester, however, having become familiar with the healthy body, the

---

1794; Representación del Colegio de San Carlos, Dec. 31, 1795; AUC, Libro de Acuerdos (1804–1810), Juntas of April 24, June 12, 1806.

On the use of wax models in general, see Thomas N. Haviland and Lawrence C. Parish, "A Brief Account of the Use of Wax Models in the Study of Medicine," *Journal of the History of Medicine and Allied Sciences*, XXV (1970), 52–75.

14. *Ordenanzas* (1787), Parte Segunda, Sec. I, Cap. III.

15. Erwin H. Ackerknecht, *A Short History of Medicine* (New York, 1955), pp. 124–125.

student was ready to study "the human body when it is sick"—pathology. Following Boerhaave, the professor identified each disease by "class, genus, and species," examined its causes and symptoms, and discussed possible cures. The course concluded with the basic principles of therapeutics.[16] Its almost Aristotelian approach suggests that Gimbernat intended the course as a rational framework on which to base more specific, practical material later. Modern scholars have criticized many eighteenth-century surgeons for being too eager to perform operations and amputations so dangerous that the patient usually died from shock or infection.[17] Therefore, the selection of Boerhaave was a sound move, for he and his students emphasized the curative powers of the body, a healthy return to Hippocratic principles.

Pathology was a new science in the late eighteenth century. Of extreme importance in light of later developments was the work of Giovanni Battista Morgagni (1682–1771). Morgagni drew a logical relationship between the results of some seven hundred autopsies and the symptoms he had observed before death. Ironically, the practicing eighteenth-century surgeon was already more familiar with pathology, at least in practice, than was the educated physician. His own experience in setting bones and treating wounds necessarily led him to relate symptoms and causes to a specific result. He felt the bone and observed the wound before deciding on treatment. Thus, the logical approach of the San Carlos course provided just the theoretical background the surgeon needed. The physician, on the other hand, was more apt to base his treatment on his abstract theory of the nature of disease. Hence, the propensity for bleedings and purges.[18]

After two years of studying the basic sciences necessary for good medical and surgical practice, the student was ready to move on to surgery itself. During the autumn of his third year he began to study surgical diseases, the specific infirmities with which he would come into direct contact. The course emphasized tumors, wounds, especially wounds from firearms, inflammations, ulcers, and maladies of the eyes, ears, and nose. These were the main concerns of surgeons at the time. Though more specific in content, the structure of the course was very similar to pathology. The instructor divided each major topic into

16. *Ordenanzas* (1787), Parte Segunda, Sec. I, Cap. III.

17. Owsei Temkin, "The Role of Surgery in the Rise of Modern Medical Thought," *Bulletin of the History of Medicine*, XXV (1951), 248–250.

18. *Ibid.*, pp. 254 ff. Temkin argues that the empirical approach of the surgeon eventually encouraged the physician to turn away from theory and adopt the surgeon's pragmatism.

"class, genus, and species," and in each case explained the causes, symptoms, prognosis and treatment. The suggested text was *Cirugía expurgada* by Johann Gorter (1689–1762), another of Boerhaave's students.[19] (The University of Salamanca had adopted the same text in its reform.)

After 1795, students repeated the course the following year. The statutes of that year also added the still-novel subject of legal medicine to the content of the course. The surgeon was becoming an important adjunct to solving crime and administering justice. The course emphasized the correct preparation of legal reports on the nature and probable cause of wounds. The treatises used were those of Pablo Zachías (1584–1659) and Johann Bohn (1640–1719), the founders of that subject.

During the second half of his third year, the student learned the other principal component of surgery, the art of setting bones and treating fractures (*algebra quirurgical*). According to the 1787 plan, the course was repeated again in the fourth year, taught by the professor of operations. After 1795 it was taught by the versatile professor of venereal disease and was not repeated. The same Gorter text was used. The separation of bone-setting from the other branches of surgery portended the gradual elimination of this less sophisticated task from the realm of surgery.

Third-year students were also introduced to obstetrics and pediatrics, two arts as old as man himself, but ones that were just becoming academically and professionally respectable by the end of the century. Individuals such as William Hunter and William Smellie[20] were offering private instruction in London, and Manchester, and were heroically trying to raise midwifery to the level of a profession. But for the most part untrained midwives continued to dominate obstetrics throughout Europe as a result of tradition and concern for modesty. Pediatrics was similarly ignored by the medical profession despite the question, how could one diagnose a child who could not describe what bothered him?[21] Before 1787 there existed no formal instruction in either subject in Spain.

19. Johannes Gorter (1689–1762) was professor of medicine at the University of Hardewijk as a result of Boerhaave's recommendation. Though a popular teacher, he did not have the prestige of many of his contemporaries. See Lindeboom, *Herman Boerhaave*, pp. 43, 225. Most general histories of medicine do not mention him.

20. William Smellie (1697–1763), Hunter's instructor in obstetrics, gave private lessons in his London home. He improved the forceps and wrote rules for their use.

21. Garrison, *An Introduction to the History of Medicine*, pp. 337–340; Ackerknecht,

Antonio Gimbernat probably became aware of the urgent need to upgrade obstetrics during his years of travel. In his first report in 1780 he mentioned the importance of adding obstetrics to the education of a surgeon.[22] His statutes of 1787 assigned a chair of obstetrics (*partos*) and venereal diseases. Those of 1795 created a separate chair of venereal disease and added bandages and bone-setting to his responsibility in a sort of a potpourri of surgical miscellany. Under the 1787 plan the student studied venereal diseases in the fall and obstetrics in the spring; in 1795 the order was reversed.[23]

The course in obstetrics covered more than childbirth. Using the relevant sections of Boerhaave and the treatises of Jean Astruc, André Levret, and others, the instructor explained "the diseases peculiar to women, those of children, and everything relevant to the obstetrical art, the knowledge of which is of so much interest to human nature."[24] In 1795 the course was extended to a full year. Luis Franceschi constructed several life-size exhibits with which instructors illustrated their lectures. Indeed, the entire concept of formal teaching in this area was a tremendous novelty in Spanish medical education.

However, Gimbernat fully realized that a few surgeons familiar with modern obstetrics would have little effect upon the tremendous loss of life associated with childbirth. Thus, he included in his plan a provision whereby the professor of obstetrics would offer free lessons in the art to interested women, a sort of extension course for the community. Only married women of pure blood could attend. Once the courses began, no woman in the Madrid area was to be licensed as a midwife by the Protomedicato without having attended them. The class itself included the function of the various female organs, signs of pregnancy, types of delivery and respective procedures, and proper care of the newborn infant.

According to the ordinances, the obstetrical instruction for both San Carlos students and midwives was scheduled to start March 1790

*A Short History of Medicine*, p. 123; Shryock, *The Development of Modern Medicine*, pp. 83–84.

22. "Informe de Gimbernat," July 14, 1780, in *Obras de Gimbernat*, II, 145–154.

23. Syphilis, one of the first diseases to be specifically identified, was one of the major health problems of the eighteenth century. It was generally treated with mercurial fumigation and inunction by a surgeon or barber. The course on it at San Carlos was undoubtedly a useful one for the future surgeon. (Garrison, *An Introduction to the History of Medicine, The Development of Modern Medicine*, pp. 12, 78.)

24. *Ordenanzas* (1787), Parte Segunda, Sec. II, Cap. I. Jean Astruc (1684–1766) wrote a six-volume treatise on gynecology. André Levret (1730–1780), an early proponent of male midwifery in Paris, wrote on delivery procedures and introduced several new instruments.

when the first class reached that point in the curriculum. The Council of Castile posted notices throughout Madrid announcing the free public instruction. The class would meet for two hours in the evening twice a week and would last two years. On April 19, formal ceremonies inaugurated the public lessons. Once again Pablo Ferrándiz of the Council of Castile presided. The students were present, two from the school and eight women who were to begin the course. Agustín Ginesta, the professor of obstetrics, gave a formal lecture on the importance of his subject.[25]

The makeshift arrangements for an obstetrical clinic illustrate the practical problems the school faced in its early years and the imaginative steps it took to solve them. Modesty demanded a special clinic isolated from the rest of the school, but none was available at the Hospital General. Accordingly, the school worked out an arrangement with the Royal House for the Abandoned (*Real Casa de los Desamparados*) whereby the professor of obstetrics could use its maternity ward as a clinic for his students. In return, the professor would assist the staff there several hours a week. The Crown was not pleased with the arrangement, but it continued for several years. At least it placed no additional financial burden on the Royal Treasury.

San Carlos also initiated a significant step for improving obstetrical care for the poor by suggesting that each of the midwives trained at San Carlos be assigned to one of the eight quarters of Madrid. There she would offer free assistance to the poor and instruction to local midwives. The Crown would pay her salary. Needless to say, such a proposal for government-supported medical care for the poor led to considerable debate. As always, money was a problem. But finally, in July 1794, the Crown agreed. A royal order asked the college to nominate the eight women. This was easily accomplished, for at that point, only eight midwives had completed the course. Funds for the program came from the recently established General Board of Welfare (*Junta General de Caridad*).[26]

The whole realm of pregnancy and childbirth was intertwined with the Catholic concern for universal baptism and the popular social

25. AFM, Libro de Representaciones, Ordenes, etc., Representación del Colegio de San Carlos, March 5, 1790; Libro de Acuerdos (1787–1804), Juntas of Feb. 25, April 15, April 19, 1790.

26. AFM, Libro de Representaciones, Ordenes, etc., Representación del Colegio de San Carlos, March 5, 1790; Informes del Colegio de San Carlos, July 12, 1791, Dec. 6, 1794; Real orden, July 13, 1794; Libro de Acuerdos (1787–1804), Juntas of March 31, 1791, July 17, July 24, 1794.

concern for feminine modesty. The course on childbirth included lessons on the proper administration of baptism in cases of emergency, including baptism of the fetus in miscarriage. All instruction was behind "closed doors." Only students in the course could accompany the professor on his clinical rounds. And in "delicate cases of secret pregnancies" or when the patient was strongly opposed to witnesses, the professor would attend to the patient without students at his side.[27]

The dual program in obstetrics was significant for several reasons. In the first place, it marked an important step in the Spanish Crown's assumption of greater responsibility for the health of its subjects. It also revealed a deep concern on the part of the San Carlos faculty for improving everyday practice. Finally, by both incorporating obstetrics into the surgical curriculum and offering special courses for practicing midwives, San Carlos endeavored to improve the practice of obstetrics without driving women out of medicine. Indeed, formal training could only raise the status of midwives, much as San Carlos had raised the status of surgery.

In the fourth year the student proceeded to the study of operations. This course included the causes and symptoms of conditions requiring an operation and a description of the surgeon's instruments. Again, demonstration and practice were the watchwords. Every student had to practice each operation on a cadaver until he could perform it perfectly. The professor followed the *Curso teórico práctico de operaciones de cirugía*, by Diego Velasco y Villaverde, a Spanish army surgeon who taught at the Barcelona college. After 1795 the professor also made frequent reference to the published *Memorias* of the Academy of Surgery of Paris. The course was repeated the following year.

Of course, the average eighteenth-century surgeon performed relatively few operations as we know them. The sophisticated accomplishments about which one reads in medical histories were usually limited to the renowned practitioner in a college or clinic. The lack of effective anesthetic restricted the surgeon and put a premium on speed. Ignorant of bacteria, surgeons little realized the importance of sterile conditions. As a result, many a successful operation was followed by the patient's dying of shock or infection. In addition, internal medicine, having little understanding of local pathology, still attributed most illnesses

27. *Ordenanzas* (1787), Parte Segunda, Sec. II, Cap. I; AFM, Libro de Representaciones, Ordenes, etc., Informe del Colegio de San Carlos, Dec. 6, 1794.

to the general condition of the body. Thus, a disease called for surgical treatment only when it was clearly related to a particular location in the body, as occurred with obstructions and stones. When a single limb became infected, the customary solution was to amputate the limb. To some extent, then, the sophisticated operative techniques the San Carlos student learned had little immediate application. Yet it was precisely this knowledge that placed the San Carlos graduate far above the romance surgeon. He was a scientist, not a craftsman.

After 1795 the fourth-year student also attended a class in botany. This science had grown rapidly in the eighteenth century. Spaniards in both public and private life were particularly enthusiastic about its possibilities; Ferdinand VI established a botanical garden and Charles III funded botanical expeditions to the New World. Since the records of San Carlos do not mention a chair of botany, students presumably attended the class offered in the Botanical Gardens.

The fifth-year student repeated the courses of the previous year and began his study of materia médica, the remedies available to the surgeon and physician. After an introduction to chemistry and the basic sources of medicines, the instructor proceeded to give the student "precise information of simple and compound remedies, their class, properties, dosage, preparation, and external application or internal administration."[28] Finally, the student learned "the art of prescribing," perhaps including a little practical psychology. The professor of materia médica was also responsible for maintaining a collection of drugs.

By now the student knew enough of surgery to begin his own practice. However, Gimbernat believed the surgeon needed a broad understanding of the healing arts as a whole, not just his own craft. Accordingly, the San Carlos men received a brief instruction of the realm of the physician. Under the 1787 statutes the student during his fifth year studied "mixed diseases," illnesses having both medical and surgical causes or remedies. The 1795 statutes, which extended the program to six years, placed this in the sixth year and more forthrightly dubbed it theoretical-practical medicine. The course, which emphasized types of fevers, followed the *Aphorisms* of Boerhaave and Hippocrates. Thus, the graduate of San Carlos knew more about internal medicine than the university medical graduate did about surgery.

By 1800 there were five colleges of surgery in Spain. In order to standardize their operation and make additional improvements, the

28. *Ibid.*, Sec. I, Cap. IV.

Crown named a commission of physicians and surgeons to draw up still another set of statutes.[29] Gimbernat, who was a member, prepared a lengthy proposal for the full commission. It differed from his previous plans in its greater emphasis on the natural sciences. Each college would have additional chairs of chemistry, botany, and physics. Gimbernat also wanted a course in comparative anatomy.

This commission, however, was not prepared to accept the advice of Gimbernat. The struggles of the past few years over the reunification of medicine and surgery had created tremendous tensions and jealousies.[30] Perhaps some members of the commission felt Gimbernat already had too much power, or thought that he had no business appropriating to his school of surgery what properly belonged to secondary education. At any rate, the commission rejected Gimbernat's proposal out of hand. The faculty of San Carlos submitted statements in support of Gimbernat. Several students even read papers in their public exercises on the utility of chemistry, but all to no avail.

The resulting ordinances of 1804, which did not radically differ from previous ones, contained several healthy innovations.[31] The time spent in the clinic was increased. The anatomy course was extended to a full year. No specific texts were assigned; instead, the individual instructor was to make his own choice with the approval of his colleagues. On the other hand, several of Gimbernat's principal contributions to surgical education—professional specialization, the need for the most recent text, the importance of a background in natural science—were missing. The ordinances provided for three "supernumerary" chairs; when a vacancy occurred, the senior substitute professor would fill it. Hence, an individual instructor was less likely to have done serious research in the particular branch of surgery he taught. In choosing a text, the professor was to favor "the classical authors who have written with such exactitude." A distinction was made between Latin and romance students. Only Latin students would continue their studies for the sixth year in which medical theory and practice were taught.

29. The only account of the commission's work is in Agustín de Gimbernat, *Noticia de Gimbernat*, pp. 52–55.

30. See Chapter VI. Medicine and surgery were legally united as one science and one profession in 1799, only to be redivided a year later.

31. AHN, Universidades, Alcalá-Cátedras, Leg. 42, Num. 74, *Real Cédula de S. M. y Señores del Consejo, en que se aprueban y mandan observar las Ordenanzas generales formadas para el régimen escolástico y económico de los Reales Colegios de Cirugía, y gobierno de esta Facultad en todo el Reyno* (Madrid, 1804). Hereinafter cited as *Ordenanzas Generales* (1804).

Worst of all, to Gimbernat, was the absence of the natural sciences. Not only were there no chairs of chemistry, physics, or botany, but the ordinances even permitted "Scholastic philosophy" in place of experimental physics as an entrance requirement. When asked to comment on this aspect of the new ordinances, Gimbernat called Scholastic philosophy "entirely useless" for the potential surgeon.[32]

Despite these modest setbacks, the San Carlos curriculum was still basically that of Antonio Gimbernat. The faculty continued to teach according to his rules, and both the curriculum itself and the principles behind it represented substantial advances in several respects. It was clearly based upon subject matter, not specific authors who could easily become out of date. Gimbernat exhibited a tremendous faith in the individual instructor to select the best material for his lectures at a time when most school statutes prescribed mandatory texts for teacher and student alike. The course itself was an organic whole in which each course led easily and rationally to the next. Indeed, the introductory program of anatomy, physiology, and pathology is still followed in most medical schools. Graduates of the school were more than craftsmen. Implicit in the curriculum was an effort to train students to think as sensitive men of science and to take their professional responsibilities seriously. Finally, the statutes placed great emphasis on effective teaching. The constant demonstrations and the daily practical experience made the difference between a learned scholar and an effective practitioner. In the final analysis, it was probably the personal experience far more than the modern texts and ordered curriculum that made the San Carlos graduate an excellent surgeon.

These factors alone would have made the College of San Carlos very modern for its day, but its crowning glory was its clinic where students had the opportunity to treat large numbers of patients on a daily basis. Indeed, the growth of clinical medical training was probably the greatest accomplishment of eighteenth-century medical education. One medical historian has associated the dawn of modern medicine with the introduction of clinical teaching.[33] "Hospital medicine," as he called it, gave the student wider experience and the opportunity to compare symptoms, diseases, and medications on a large scale. The course of an illness could be carefully followed from begin-

32. Quoted in Agustín de Gimbernat, *Noticia de Gimbernat*, pp. 54–55.

33. Ackernecht, *A Short History of Medicine*, pp. 133–136. See also his *Medicine at the Paris Hospital*, esp. pp. xi–xiii.

ning to end; if a patient died, an autopsy could provide still additional knowledge.

Gimbernat was determined to make clinical instruction an essential part of the San Carlos curriculum from the start. He envisioned a large clinic of some forty patients with separate wards for men and women. Students of the third year and beyond would spend most of their time in the clinic. San Carlos professors would choose which patients would be admitted to the clinic and be responsible for their treatment. Twelve resident students (*colegiales internos*) would assist in caring for the patient and, in return, receive free room and board plus a small stipend of five reales a day.[34]

Unfortunately, obtaining a clinic was not so easily accomplished in practice. Early in the 1789–1790 academic year the school petitioned for a clinic so that the third-year students "might see the rules and axioms of their various professors verified in practice at the head of a patient's bed," as provided in the ordinances.[35] In January the Council of Castile requested additional details. The response clearly indicated the reduced hopes the school had by this time. It meekly suggested a small clinic of six to eight patients; any hospital would do. Perhaps a larger clinic would be possible when the school moved into permanent quarters.[36] Nothing further occurred for several months. It was beyond the authority of the school to take over a clinic on its own, and it lacked the funds to provide the stipend for the resident students. Meanwhile, the students were missing valuable experience. Apparently the cool relationship between the school and the Hospital General worsened the situation.

In mid-August several members of the Council, the administrators of the Hospital General, and Antonio Gimbernat and Mariano Rivas held a series of informal meetings to arrange the details for a clinic in the Hospital General. The college and the hospital both tried to profit from the arrangement and at a minimum cost. According to the final agreement, San Carlos would choose the patients for the clinic with an eye toward the educational value of their disease. The college would be completely responsible for providing medical personnel, administer-

34. *Ordenanzas* (1787), Parte Tercera; "Informe de Gimbernat," July 14, 1780, in *Obras de Gimbernat*, II, 145–154.

35. AFM, Libro de Representaciones, Ordenes, etc., Representación del Colegio de San Carlos, Nov. 6, 1789.

36. *Ibid.*, Orden del Consejo, Jan. 14, 1790; Informe del Colegio de San Carlos, Jan. 29, 1790.

ing medications, and changing sheets and clothing. The hospital would pay for the patients' meals and medicines. It would also nominate a senior intern (*practicante mayor*), to be paid by the college, who would supervise the patients' daily care. Finally, San Carlos would provide free advice to the hospital personnel upon request. The Crown approved the arrangements on condition that they entail no additional cost to the Royal Treasury. The rooms were finally ready to receive patients in December 1790. Gimbernat himself prepared a set of rules for the students to follow.[37]

Still the clinic did not open for another two and one-half years. The first class graduated with no clinical experience. The responsibility for this delay seems to have been the result of further bickering over finances and the usual sluggish pace of the Spanish bureaucracy. Since the money for the resident students had been appropriated for the senior intern of the hospital, the school petitioned the Crown for additional funds. The tedious consultations and referrals for additional advice pursued their course. Finally, in July 1793, the Crown agreed to supply the needed money from the Royal Lottery. The clinic formally opened the following month.[38]

Eighteenth-century clinical instruction did not use an entire hospital for its laboratory. Instead, a small number of patients were chosen, housed in a separate facility, and cared for by the instructional staff. Nevertheless, a contemporary medical student would probably feel quite at home in the San Carlos clinic. Patients were carefully selected so that their illness would fit in well with what was being taught. The professors were especially eager to find unique cases. No doubt the patients were delighted to have been chosen, since they received expert care and each had his own bed. At eight in the morning and four in the afternoon (three-thirty in winter) one of the professors, accompanied by several students, visited each patient. He pointed out the particular illness and its symptoms, what remedies he was using, and any changes in the patient's condition. Each student was assigned to keep a detailed diary of one of the patients, noting any change in appearance, diet, temperature, even weather conditions. In 1805 the school purchased a thermometer and a barometer to make daily read-

37. *Ibid.*, Ordenes del Consejo, Sept. 16, Sept. 17, 1790; AFM, Libro de Acuerdos (1787–1804), Juntas of Sept. 24, Oct. 7, Dec. 9, 1790.

38. AFM, Libro de Representaciones, Ordenes, etc., Representación del Colegio de San Carlos, Feb. 14, July 12, 1791; Real orden, July 24, 1793.

ings readily available.[39] Such a detailed study of the course of one patient was a valuable lesson in showing that disease was a developing phenomenon, not a static one. It also taught the student the merit of accurate observation, perseverance, and patience.

The eight resident students received still additional experience. Most had studied two years before receiving their appointments. Each resident took a turn at being in attendance at the clinic twenty-four hours a day. The residents were also responsible for changing sheets and clothing, giving medication, and all the other menial tasks associated with hospital care. No doubt it was an exhausting but valuable experience. After 1795 the resident students received their title of Latin surgeon without charge. They had most certainly earned it.

Of course, the clinic also created disciplinary problems. Most students spent far less time in the clinic than their professors would have liked, and some frequently missed the morning and afternoon visits. On one occasion the junta warned that repeated absences could prevent a student from taking his exams. Even the resident students could be troublesome. Often their work was sloppy and their behavior boisterous. One student lost his stipend because of "bad conduct" in the infirmary after repeated warnings. The proximity to the hospital was also a nuisance. Pupils would wander through the hospital, strangers would wander through the school, and sometimes patients from the hospital used the school as a convenient way to make an unnoticed escape from the hospital. In 1807 a lock was placed on the door connecting the two.[40]

Such minor nuisances did not invalidate clinical training. Indeed, a similar clinic was established for medical students in 1795. For the first time medicine imitated the methods of surgery.

The College of San Carlos was governed by its faculty, who met as the administrative and academic junta (*Junta Gubernativa y Escolástica*) every Thursday. The junta was responsible for managing the school's finances, making all appointments not subject to the oposición, certifying students for graduation, and, in general, supervising the day-to-day operation of the school. The rigid statutes of the school severely restricted its flexibility, however, and the faculty was reluctant to deviate from established procedures without permission. Such tight

39. AUC, Libro de Acuerdos (1804–1810), Junta of April 18, 1805. The general description is based on AFM, Libro de Representaciones, Ordenes, etc., Orden del Consejo, Sept. 16, 1790, and the ordenanzas of 1789, 1795, and 1804.

40. Such incidents were common. See, for example, AUC, Libro de Acuerdos (1804–1810), Juntas of Sept. 11, 1804; Feb. 5, Oct. 8, 1807.

controls were not surprising, of course, since the Crown was determined to have all education under its firm control. As a result, the school was constantly petitioning the Crown to grant exceptions to the rules in certain cases.

Most of the business of the San Carlos junta was routine—whether a student should get credit for a course, how a disciplinary problem might be solved, what answer a royal inquiry should receive, which students should be admitted or appointed to assist in the clinic, whether to give a professor or student permission to travel during the academic year. When public disasters occurred, such as a 1790 fire in the Plaza Mayor, the school was expected to contribute to the relief effort. Most problems, however minute, had to be referred to higher authorities for a final decision. As a result, the junta spent most of its meetings preparing petitions and responding to edicts.

As a further restriction upon its autonomy, an appointee of the Crown always possessed ultimate authority over San Carlos. The ordinances of 1787 gave this authority to the First Surgeon of the king, naming him president of the school. The president was obliged to consult with the junta before taking action, but he could veto any of its decisions. Pedro Custodio Gutiérrez, who had suggested a school of surgery in 1768, was automatically the first president by virtue of being the king's First Surgeon. Antonio Gimbernat and Mariano Rivas, who had actually created the school, were the co-directors. As such they alternately presided over official functions but had no other power.

From the start there was considerable friction between Gimbernat and Custodio Gutiérrez. The two men had had bitter disagreements over the nature of the school; cooperation between them became virtually nonexistent. In 1790 they engaged in an ugly dispute over salaries. Custodio Gutiérrez felt his four thousand reales salary was not in accord with the prestige of his office since professors received eighteen thousand reales. The school, led by Gimbernat, strongly opposed any increase, even though the government, not the school, would have paid it. With perhaps a little jealousy, the junta reminded the Crown of the income its president received from his other duties and righteously observed that the professors devoted all their efforts to the school.[41] In 1795 Custodio Gutiérrez hesitated in appointing a director to replace Gimbernat. Again the junta was moved to angry

41. AFM, Libro de Representaciones, Ordenes, etc., Informe del Colegio de San Carlos, April 8, 1790.

remonstrances.[42] Even death could not heal the wounds. In 1801 the school received a request to list the accomplishments (*méritos*) of Custodio Gutiérrez for his eulogy. Manuel Bonafos, the school's librarian, replied that he had no record of any.[43]

Perhaps Gimbernat simply disliked sharing authority over "his school," for he also engaged in several controversies with his co-director, Mariano Rivas. In 1793 Rivas voted not to accept and approve Gimbernat's paper on his crural hernia operation. In 1795 Rivas was not promoted with the other senior professors. Finally, the Crown gave him a pension as Surgeon of the Bedchamber but removed him from the San Carlos post he had held "in perpetuity."[44]

Internal discord helped hasten the demise of San Carlos's semi-autonomy. In April 1795 the Crown created a Superior Administrative Board (*Junta Superior Gubernativa*) to supervise all colleges of surgery, citing "the continual discord among the personnel of the Royal Colleges of Surgery" as one of the reasons.[45] Although San Carlos professors would dominate the board, the school found itself more constrained than ever.

From the very beginning the professors of San Carlos constantly endeavored to boost the prestige of the college, and, therefore, of surgery itself. In 1789, after several petitions, the Crown permitted future graduates of San Carlos to enter an oposición for a chair of anatomy in any university. Six years later the school received the right to grant its own bachelor of arts degree.[46] Lesser matters also occupied the professors' attention. In the early years much correspondence concerned the need for a school seal. Later the professors established a fund for widows and children of faculty members. In 1791, frustrated at the lack of response from the Inquisition, the professors even petitioned Rome directly for permission to read prohibited books.

During the 1790s the Crown was engaged in reforming the requirements and procedures for obtaining a license to practice surgery. A cédula of 1797 declared that all potential romance surgeons in the Madrid area would have to attend San Carlos for three years as audi-

42. AFM, Libro de Acuerdos (1787–1804), Junta of July 14, 1795.

43. *Ibid.*, Junta of Oct. 8, 1801.

44. *Ibid.*, Junta of April 11, 1793; AFM, Libro de Representaciones, Ordenes, etc., Reales ordenes, April 19, May 4, 1795.

45. AFM, Libro de Representaciones, Ordenes, etc., Real orden, April 19, 1795. External regulation of the profession is discussed in the following chapter.

46. *Ibid.*, Representación del Colegio de San Carlos, Nov. 3, 1789; AFM, Libro de Acuerdos para la Junta Superior, Orden de la Junta Superior, Oct. 10, 1795.

tors.[47] Immediately the college faced an influx of ill-prepared students for whom a curriculum had to be formed. The junta hurriedly set up a course in which the romance students would attend the classes of anatomy, surgical diseases, wound dressings, venereal diseases and obstetrics, and operations. However, the professors expressed doubt that such a three-year condensed course was really adequate.[48]

In 1804 the junta received the far greater burden of administering the licensing examinations. The new statutes of that year granted the colleges of surgery the exclusive right to grant licenses to practice surgery throughout Spain. Moreover, all surgeons had to attend one of the colleges in order to be eligible for examination for a license. Surgery had now completed its difficult transition from a trade to a profession.

Years of study, not years of apprenticeship, were now the prerequisite to becoming a surgeon. Except for obstetrics and bleeding, one could not practice any branch of the healing arts in Spain without formal academic training. This was not only a radical departure from the Spanish past but put Spain into the forefront of progressive medical legislation. In France, by contrast, one could become an *officier de santé* with only an apprenticeship and examination until 1892.[49] Ironically, these progressive regulations maintained the many traditional distinctions within the surgical profession. And since a baptismal certificate and proof of "pure blood" were still required for matriculation, they remained prerequisites for practicing surgery.

In entrusting the responsibility of granting licenses to the colleges of surgery, the Crown broke with the long-standing Spanish tradition of separating an academic degree from a legal license to practice. Each school now made the final decision on the competency of its own graduates to practice surgery. The new responsibility also drastically changed the nature of the schools. Originally they were small, highly selective institutions designed to train the future leaders of the profession. A graduate would one day receive a distinguished appointment and perhaps engage in research or become a teacher himself. Now the

47. AHN, Consejos, Leg. 1845, Exp. 10, Real cédula . . . en que se prescribe el Método que ha de observarse en el Tribunal de Proto-Cirujanato en los exámenes de Cirujanos . . . , May 12, 1797. Also *Nov. Rec.*, VIII, xii, 4.

48. AFM, Libro de Acuerdos para la Junta Superior, Representación del Colegio de San Carlos, May 4, 1797.

49. Ackerknecht, *Medicine at the Paris Hospital*, p. 39. The French Revolution destroyed the distinction between physician and surgeon and created a general practitioner known as an *officier de santé.*

schools had become mandatory for every surgeon. While the ability of the average practitioner increased, the academic level of the classes themselves probably fell. Classes increased in size and students had less opportunity for individual practice and experiment. The student body was divided into a large number of romance students and a small minority of favored Latin students. It was as if a small, selective, private college suddenly became a large state university, but continued to admit students of high ability who paid their own way and received a superior education.

The problems of licensing also became the main preoccupation of the weekly meetings of the junta. Not only were the licensing examinations themselves extremely time-consuming, but there were innumerable cases that required special consideration. Could a man be licensed if he lacked one course, or had taken it out of order? What if he changed schools, or had studied abroad? Could he count the years of practice before he entered the college? Could he change from romance to Latin, or vice versa? Could he apply a previously paid fee to this examination? The problems seemed infinite. And the junta found more and more of its time taken up with making fine legal decisions. The minutes of the weekly meetings became far more voluminous after 1804, though pedagogical and scientific questions came up less frequently.[50]

In addition, the junta of San Carlos suddenly became responsible for handling large amounts of money. The statutes were always especially detailed on financial matters. In the absence of banks and checking accounts, the junta was charged with guaranteeing the physical security of the school's funds. For this purpose, it kept the money in the classic chest with three locks. The director, the secretary, and one professor each had a key that opened one of the locks. At the last meeting of the year the junta prepared a financial report on that year. The junta was extremely diligent in keeping accurate financial records, noting every expense from purchases of chairs and paper to repairing the school clock and printing notices.

During the early years the finances of the school were relatively simple.[51] The Crown gave the school eighteen thousand reales per year.

50. The Libros de Acuerdos testify to this shift of attention and the time-consuming nature of handling licensing. One example is the books themselves, all physically the same size. The first volume (1787–1804) covers fourteen years, but no other volume covers more than six.

51. Financial data are based on AFM, Libro de Cuentas (1786–1815); AUC, Contabilidad-Salidas de Caudales, 1791–1820 (hereinafter cited as AUC, Contabilidad [1791–1820]). The former is an account book with a running balance; the latter lists only expenses, but in more detail.

This sum was more than adequate for slowly expanding the library and exhibit and for paying current expenses. The school charged its students nothing. In 1796 it began to receive additional income from the Royal Lottery to help pay the resident students their daily stipend. Both figures wavered between 20,000 and 25,000 reales. However, after 1797, the annual subsidy began to decline.

After 1801 the finances of San Carlos became more complex, for now it was entrusted with the funds for all the surgical colleges. It was responsible for paying all salaries and purchasing all equipment for five colleges. The royal subsidy dropped sharply; by 1804 the colleges as a whole were almost self-supporting. The dramatic change became possible because the colleges now conducted examinations for licenses and collected the respective fees. The annual fees for licenses amounted to more than 350,000 reales for all of Spain. Thus, the assumption of licensing duties by the colleges not only increased student enrollment and consumed much of the professors' time but also gave the schools financial independence. Though some government support was still needed from time to time to make ends meet, the very existence of San Carlos was no longer dependent upon royal largess.

To most San Carlos professors, however, the burdensome details of administration were probably an unwelcome distraction from their primary task of training future surgeons. Indeed, the principal asset of the college was its dedicated teachers. Most professors had held important posts in a military or civilian hospital before beginning their career of teaching.[52] Many had also studied at one of the colleges of surgery themselves. Indeed, three of San Carlos's first dozen students later joined its faculty, and the custom continued. Some had studied outside of Spain and others had received royal honors. A good number carried on important research or published monographs and classroom texts. During the early years a disproportionately large number of the faculty came from Catalonia.

A chair at San Carlos was a lucrative position. Every professor received an annual salary of eighteen thousand reales. (San Carlos professors received six thousand reales more than their colleagues in the other surgical colleges in order to meet the higher cost of living in Madrid.) In addition, twenty reales of every licensing examination fee went to each examining professor. And, looking to the future, a professor at San Carlos could reasonably expect to receive additional

52. Alvarez-Sierra, *Historia de la cirugía española*, gives biographical sketches of the early San Carlos faculty.

honors and, perhaps, a lucrative pension. Thus, financial factors supplemented the excellent reputation of San Carlos in attracting an outstanding faculty.[53]

Partly as a result of its excellence, the San Carlos faculty was remarkably unstable. By 1795 only five of the original professors were still teaching; by 1802 none of these remained.[54] In addition to expected retirement and deaths, many faculty members received royal titles such as Surgeon of the Royal Bedchamber with their accompanying pension. Most members of the Superior Board of Surgery were former San Carlos instructors who vacated their posts at the college.

Professors won their appointment either by royal order, as did the original faculty members in 1787, or by oposición. Until 1804 each professor received an appointment to a specific chair. If he resigned, the Crown often assigned his professorship to another faculty member. The dissector was often promoted in this manner. However, the ordinances of 1804 divided the faculty into nine regular chairs (*cátedras de número*), each of which was assigned a specific course, and three substitute chairs. When a chair became vacant, the senior substitute professor automatically filled it and was himself replaced by oposición. Substitute professors received an annual salary of twelve thousand reales and fully participated in all academic exercises.[55] The new procedure facilitated the transition and eliminated long vacancies and the need to juggle instructors from one chair to another, but it also destroyed the specialization Gimbernat believed was so important.

Most professors earned their position by the oposición, an academic ritual with a long tradition in Spanish higher education that exists in modified form even today. The statutes of the college provided detailed instructions for carrying out the oposición with which the junta carefully complied. Much of the correspondence between the junta and

53. It is difficult and hazardous to try to determine the value of eighteenth-century monetary amounts. Other salaries within San Carlos provide some basis for comparison. Luis Franceschi, who made the anatomical exhibits, earned 6,600 reales a year. The *portero* earned only 1,200 reales, plus board.

The Appendix of Hamilton, *War and Prices in Spain*, provides figures for further comparisons. A master cabinetmaker, by far the best paid craftsman listed, earned some 6,000 reales a year (six days per week, fifty-two weeks a year), assuming steady employment—a hazardous assumption. An unskilled laborer, using the same assumptions, earned only 1,560 reales a year. Food prices offer another possible basis for comparison. With his monthly pay a San Carlos professor could purchase 500 dozen eggs. Assuming eggs sell today for about 90¢ per dozen, this would be the rough equivalent of $450.

54. All arrivals and departures are duly noted in the Libros de Acuerdos.

55. *Ordenanzas Generales* (1804), Cap. V.

higher governing authorities concerned minor variations made necessary by unforeseen circumstances. New statutes made no substantial changes.

In essence, the oposición was a contest for a vacant position. Each candidate tried to outdo his competitors in delivering learned lectures in Latin, answering questions with wit and confidence in the same language, and displaying his competence as a surgeon. It was a grueling experience for the *opositor*, though perhaps as good a means as any for choosing the most competent man for a position.

The procedure was initiated when the Council of Castile (Superior Board after 1795) gave formal permission to the school to post placards announcing the vacancy and named three professors to serve as judges (*censores*) in the competition.[56] San Carlos then sent posters to all colleges of surgery, to all universities, and to the major cities. In turn, it frequently received similar announcements from other colleges and universities. A typical announcement described the duties of the particular vacant chair, the reason for the vacancy, the salary, and the nature of the competitive exercises. It concluded with an invitation to all Latin surgeons to forward their credentials to the school and to appear for the oposición at a given time. During the first years of the college about four men usually applied for each vacant chair. As time went on the number of applicants averaged around ten. The credentials submitted by each candidate usually included a personal testament and certification from schools and licensing agencies.

Like the faculty itself, most candidates came from surgical practice rather than from academic institutions. Many held positions in the army or navy, as might be expected, since the schools prior to San Carlos were founded to train military surgeons. During the 1790s most applicants were graduates of the Barcelona college. Prospective professors apparently believed any honor would help their cause. In the oposiciones following the establishment of the doctorate, virtually every candidate claimed he was a doctor of surgery despite the fact that the degree signified no academic accomplishment. Many times the list of candidates included the names of men who had been un-

56. The following account of the oposición is based on AUC, Libro de Oposiciones-Cátedras, Vol. I; AHN, Consejos, Leg. 1285, Exp. 4, Parte 1, Expediente . . . sobre Provisión de la Cátedra de Afectos Chirúrgicos, 1789; *Ordenanzas* (1789), Parte Segunda, Sec. IV. The Libro de Oposiciones contains minute details, including a list of all topics, but stops in 1798.

All functions attributed to the Council were performed by the Superior Board after 1795 unless otherwise noted.

successful in previous oposiciones, even though the previous vacancy had been in a different area of surgery. Often a man would be successful in his second or third attempt for a position. This practice did not hurt the quality of the faculty, however, since most opositores were qualified for the position. The practice does suggest, though, that most professors had not restricted themselves to one branch of surgery before coming to San Carlos.

On the day before the date set for the first exercise of the oposición, all the candidates met in the school to draw lots for their *coopositores*, the two adversaries who would criticize their presentations. The selection was arranged in such a way that the coopositor of one candidate did not necessarily have that candidate as his own coopositor. At this point in the ritual, the applicants' credentials aslo received final approval.

The first exercise, conducted completely in Latin, began the next day. All the candidates and judges gathered in the school auditorium. In the front of the room was a large urn in which the judges had placed slips of paper, each of which contained a topic for a lecture. There were four times as many topics as there were opositores. The first candidate then approached the urn and drew three topics. After examining them, he chose one for his lecture and returned the other two to the urn without announcing them. He gave a copy of the topic he had chosen to his two coopositores. The opositor then went into seclusion in the library for twenty-four hours to prepare his lecture on the selected topic. The school provided him with a secretary and with any books he wanted. He also received a bed, meals, and refreshments, the latter consisting of bread, wine, chocolate, and ice.[57] The scholar was forbidden to speak to anyone except his secretary during the twenty-four hours.

The following day the opositor read his lecture in a formal public assembly. The length varied according to the subject. After he finished, his two coopositores had an opportunity to raise objections, point out errors, or ask questions. The competitive atmosphere easily led to some bitter exchanges. That afternoon the next candidate chose his topic in the same way.

After all the candidates had delivered their Latin lecture, the second exercise began. The procedure was exactly the same, but this time the topic, lecture, and objections were in Spanish. No doubt the spontane-

57. AFM, Libro de Cuentas (1786–1815). The two oposiciones held in 1789 cost the school almost 500 reales.

ous exchanges became both more fluent and heated in the competitors' native tongue.

The topics prepared by the judges covered the full range of surgical practice. Although the ordinances of 1787 specified that the Spanish titles were to be unrelated to the specific chair under discussion, in practice they usually were related. The topics ranged from broad expositions of general diseases to specific techniques. Topics in the oposición for the chair of obstetrics, for example, included types of deliveries, specific instruments, and signs of pregnancy. The future professor of materia médica lectured in Latin on a specific chemical. Perhaps the most varied themes were those drawn up for the chair of physiology and hygiene. They included the effects of tobacco, what places were best suited for establishing villages, the medical value of chocolate, the relation between diet and climate, even "the influence of the passions of the soul upon the human body."

The third and final exercise took place in private, with only the judges and the opositores in attendance. This time the judges personally questioned the candidate. Frequently they had the candidate perform a dissection or operate on a cadaver. The candidate was not aware of the questions in advance, though the examination often began with errors he had made in his formal presentation. The interrogation went on until the judges were satisfied with the candidate's knowledge and competence. Only the judges and the opositor himself participated. The other candidates merely listened, perhaps breathing a little easier if the opositor made some glaring error. In 1798 the school requested permission to exclude the other candidates from this oral examination. Errors were inevitable, the petition declared, and it was better that they not become public. It was unlikely that the candidates would "exercise so fraternal a respect for each other" that they would conceal each other's mistakes, and it would be embarrassing for a foolish statement of a future professor to become public knowledge. The Superior Board, by now composed entirely of former San Carlos faculty members, denied the request, ordering that the issue not be brought up again.[58] Public examinations were the only guarantee of fairness.

Finally the oposición was finished. Each judge submitted his vote and a written comment to the president of the college, who forwarded them to the Council of Castile. The Council made the final decision on who

58. AFM, Libro de Representaciones, Ordenes, etc., Representación del Colegio de San Carlos, Nov. 1798; Real orden, Dec. 12, 1798. The Crown followed the recommendation of the Superior Board.

had won the chair. After 1795 the junta of the school made the final decision. It usually concurred with the judges' decision with little debate.

The position of anatomical dissector was filled through an oposición especially designed for that post. Instead of the lecture and oral examination, the dissector had to prepare three lessons on a cadaver, one each on muscles, nerves, and the full skeleton. The procedure was similar: he pulled three topics from an urn, chose one, and had twenty-four hours in the sala de práctica to prepare the lesson.

San Carlos held its first oposición in 1789 to fill the vacant chair of obstetrics. It proceeded uneventfully, except for the long interval between the death of the previous professor and the final appointment of the next. Jaime Respau, who had held the chair since the opening of the school in 1787, died in September 1788. Announcements of the coming oposición went out in January 1789. The exercises themselves took place during April, and the Council made its final decision on July 8, almost a full year after the vacancy had occurred.

The next oposición, for the chair of surgical diseases, spawned several notable controversies that tell us much of the mentality of the early professors of San Carlos. The first concerned one of the four applicants. Joseph Barles y Alcay held a bachelor's degree in medicine and had received his license to practice surgery from a "college" in Saragossa that had received its charter from Ferdinand and Isabella. However, his license did not specify Latin surgeon. In his application, Barles y Alcay argued that it was the equivalent of a Latin surgeon's license and that he had spent most of his life teaching surgery. The junta of San Carlos agreed that the applicant was, indeed, a Latin surgeon for all practical purposes. Nevertheless, it denied him permission to enter the oposición because it did not want to set a precedent for not following the statutes precisely; it further suggested he get the proper license in Madrid.[59]

The second dispute concerned the use and significance of Latin—and the conflicting concept of the school of Antonio Gimbernat on the one hand and Mariano Rivas and Pedro Custodio Gutiérrez on the other. The specific issue was whether the objections and responses immediately following the Latin lecture could be in Spanish instead of Latin as the statutes required. On May 14, immediately preceding the exercises,

59. AUC, Libro de Oposiciones, contains the full text of this correspondence. The Royal and Imperial College of Physicians and Surgeons of Saragossa, the college in question, was most likely more of a guild that offered some instruction than a formal academic institution.

the junta discussed the problem. Gimbernat was not present, and Rivas led the argument for using Spanish. In the first oposición the exchanges had been in Latin, he argued, but there were opositores who, "though well instructed in surgery, could only speak Latin in such a confused and unclear manner that the judges and audience were mortified in the extreme." Conscious of "the disagreeable memory" of that occasion, the junta decided to allow the exchange in Spanish. This way a capable surgeon not fluent in Latin would not be at such a disadvantage. And so the objections and responses after the first oposición were in Spanish.[60]

When Gimbernat returned in July he was outraged at the change. He claimed the decision made in May was invalid because it violated the ordinances and because he had not been present. Furthermore, he demanded that the entire oposición be repeated, this time in Latin. San Carlos was an institution of Latin surgeons. Latin was important, the key to "the precious treasures of Antiquity." More to the point, all the universities and the Barcelona college conducted their oposiciones in Latin. Surely San Carlos was their equal.[61]

At any rate, the entire oposición was repeated. José Rivas y Mayor, the first opositor, gave a fine dissertation in Latin. Then his *coopositor*, José Severo López, stood up and made some telling objections in Spanish. The three judges, Pedro Custodio Gutiérrez, Antonio Fernández Solano, and Gimbernat became embroiled in a heated argument while the two opositores shouted back and forth at each other. Severo López and the third opositor argued that no one could speak in Latin extemporaneously. Rivas angrily retorted that he could. "That is just so much vanity," Custodio Gutiérrez snidely observed. Severo López made a few more points in Spanish.

The next day, with tempers still heated, it was Severo López's turn to speak. After the contestant finished, Custodio Gutiérrez, whose sympathies clearly lay with the speaker this time, allowed him a long rest. Then José Rivas rose to make an objection in Latin. He viciously criticized the speaker's "method of speaking," no doubt a reference to his less than perfect Latin. Severo López then said his manner of speech was not a proper subject of criticism. Rivas answered that it was. Custodio Gutiérrez told Rivas to sit down and keep still.[62]

During the next month the Council of Castile received arguments

60. AHN, Consejos, Leg. 1285, Exp. 4, Parte 1, Informe de Mariano Rivas, Aug. 10, 1789.

61. *Ibid.*, Informe de Antonio Gimbernat, July 21, 1789.

62. *Ibid.*, Informe de Antonio Gimbernat, Aug. 11, 1789; AUC, Libro de Oposiciones.

from both sides. Gimbernat argued that the prestige of San Carlos was at stake. If Spanish responses were allowed today, Spanish lectures would be allowed tomorrow. And then romance surgeons, the very practitioners who had destroyed Spanish surgery, would slowly take over the school. All the efforts to raise the level of Spanish surgery would go for naught. Mariano Rivas argued that San Carlos should not "perpetuate the obsolete customs of the universities." The use of Latin made language ability, not surgical ability, the key to an academic chair.

The arguments became personal as Custodio Gutiérrez and Gimbernat once again attacked each other. Both Custodio Gutiérrez and Fernández Solano, the second judge, voted for Severo López. He was well qualified, though less than adept in Latin. Gimbernat voted for Rivas. He was far superior to Severo López, who had dealt only in vague generalities. Besides, Custodio Gutiérrez had nodded his agreement to some of the latter's statements.

The Council, following the vote of the majority, approved Severo López, but the Crown overruled the Council, and Rivas received the appointment.[63] Gimbernat's personal influence at court was still high. Ten years later Severo López also joined the faculty. One wonders whether the wounds had healed.

In addition to the professors and the anatomical dissector, the statutes of San Carlos provided for a secretary and a librarian. Gimbernat had envisioned professors filling these positions for extra pay, but in 1789 the Crown assigned an army surgeon it had pensioned, Joaquín Villalva, to take charge of the library. The ordinances of 1804 assigned the duties of dissector, secretary, and librarian to the three substitute professors.[64]

The main duty of the secretary was to maintain the records of junta meetings, matriculations, and licenses. His minutes duly noted the actions taken by the meetings but without flourish. He never attributed specific arguments to specific individuals and never recorded a vote.

The librarian was responsible for the library itself and for the collection of surgical instruments. In addition, it was his duty to maintain

63. AHN, Consejos, Leg. 1285, Exp. 4, Parte 1, Expediente . . . sobre Provisión de la Cátedra de Afectos Chirúrgicos, 1789, contains all the reports and the final decisions. Whatever his reasons, Gimbernat made a wise choice. Rivas was later one of the school's most prolific writers.

64. *Ordenanzas* (1787), Parte Quinta, Sec. II; *Ordenanzas Generales* (1804), Parta Quinta; AFM, Libro de Representaciones, Ordenes, etc., Reales ordenes, Nov. 24, Dec. 29, 1789.

communications with other medical and surgical schools and academies both in Spain and abroad. The position required a fluency in Latin, French, Italian, and English.

San Carlos existed, of course, primarily for the benefit of its students. And finding qualified, motivated students proved to be one of the greatest problems the college faced during its infancy. Only three students matriculated the first year, although four others had applied. All four lacked the necessary background in the sciences, though two were licensed surgeons and the other two were licensed physicians.[65] It is ironic that the requirements of the Protomedicato for a license to practice medicine were more easily met than the requirements for matriculation at San Carlos. Only one new student matriculated in each of the following academic years. Indeed, by the end of the 1793–1794 academic year, a total of only twelve students had entered the new school. Two of these never completed the course.[66]

Nevertheless, since the classes were open to the public, they were not as empty as these figures would suggest. The classes were particularly popular the first year when up to seventy auditors attended a specific class. More than twenty of these faithfully completed the whole first-year course. Among them were prospective students still seeking to fulfill the entrance requirements, interns in the Hospital General, practicing surgeons, and "curious individuals."[67] As time went on and the school became less a novelty the number of auditors dropped, except in the anatomy lectures. Yet Gimbernat could proudly note that applicants appearing before the Protomedicato often gave answers they had heard as auditors in San Carlos.[68]

The early graduates did well. Many won appointments at army hospitals. One became a Surgeon of the Royal Family. Carlos Gimbernat, son of the director, studied in England and Scotland after completing his fourth year.[69] Four of these early students later won chairs at San Carlos. This pattern of success for the Latin graduates of the school would continue.

Enrollment climbed slowly until 1797 when graduation from San Carlos became a prerequisite to becoming a Latin surgeon. Overnight

65. AFM, Libro de Representaciones, Ordenes, etc., Informe del Colegio de San Carlos, April 10, 1788.

66. AUC, Libro de Matrícula de Cirujanos Latinos (1787–1817).

67. AFM, Libro de Representaciones, Ordenes, etc., Informe del Colegio de San Carlos, Feb. 21, 1789.

68. *Ibid.*, Informe del Colegio de San Carlos, Dec. 6, 1794.

69. *Ibid.*

the school changed from a selective institution training only those who sought an exceptional education to an essential part of Spanish higher education. By the first decade of the nineteenth century the number of Latin students alone matriculating each year averaged close to twenty, each class larger than the last.[70] Romance students probably quadrupled this number.

Such rapid growth undoubtedly changed the nature of the school. There were now as many as fifty students in a class, besides auditors. The more advanced classes were less affected because more and more students failed courses or left the school without finishing.[71] Nevertheless, only the residents who assisted in the clinic now had the personal relation with the professors that every student enjoyed in the early years.

Approximately one-third of the students who entered San Carlos completed the course. The reasons others had for dropping out varied. Some decided on another career. Others ran out of money or fell ill. If a student missed classes because of illness, he needed permission of the Superior Board to receive credit for what he had missed. Other students were expelled because they missed too many classes for no good reason. Such decisions were made on an individual basis.[72]

Every San Carlos student had to pass an oral examination at the completion of every academic year in order to pass on to the next. During the early 1800s close to half the students failed and had to repeat the year. Some simply withdrew.[73] The high proportion of failures was not surprising, for there was no test of competence before a student matriculated. Anyone who had taken the prescribed courses was admitted. Since San Carlos was a prerequisite for a license, many ill-prepared students apparently decided to give the school a try.

Students who, by royal order, received credit from other institutions were especially troublesome. In 1806, for example, the Crown decreed that San Carlos was to admit all interns from the Hospital General and credit them with the years they had spent there. In the first examination period that followed, most of the new students failed, having been found "absolutely ignorant." Fearing their ignorance might reflect on the reputation of the school, the faculty even asked that all future interns be denied advanced status. The Superior Board denied the

70. AUC, Libro de Matrícula de Cirujanos Latinos (1787–1817).

71. AUC, Libro de Matrículas Generales (1801–1805).

72. AUC, Libro de Aucerdos (1804–1810), Juntas of Oct. 4, Oct. 10, Oct. 11, Nov. 31, 1804, provides illustration of the way they reached decisions.

73. AUC, Libro de Matrícula de Cirujanos Latinos (1787–1817).

request; each case was to be considered on its own merits.[74] At any rate, the advanced training offered at San Carlos was clearly not typical of what most surgeons received.

With such an open admission policy, annual examinations would seem to have been an obvious necessity. In fact, however, such a policy was due only to the foresight of Antonio Gimbernat. In most Spanish higher education a student had only to attend a class; the only examinations were those for an academic degree. Fortunately, Gimbernat realized that an advanced course would have little value for a student who had not completely mastered its prerequisite, and so he provided in the statutes for regular examinations. The examinations themselves were formal affairs, held in September. Each student appeared before three professors and received a grade of "excellent," "passed," or "failed."[75] There was no fee for the examination.

Although the total enrollment grew, San Carlos lost many of its best students to the wars that followed the French Revolution and the rise of Napoleon. The Crown was seldom scrupulous in enforcing all the requirements for graduation when a student had joined the military. During the 1793–1794 war with France, for example, José Abades, an outstanding student, became an army surgeon in Mallorca after completing only four years. The Crown exempted him from the requirement to complete the fifth year and licensed him a Latin surgeon.[76] Other volunteers received similar dispensations.

By 1805 students were frequently serving in military hospitals before completing their studies. Frequent edicts required San Carlos to excuse them from the annual examinations and to preserve the positions of the resident students who had left. By 1807 it was difficult to find competent students to work in the clinic. For a time nonresident students worked on a day-to-day basis as none of them were fully qualified for the permanent position.[77] Such problems testify not only to the disruption created by the wars but also to the lack of outstanding students now attending the college.

74. AUC, Libro de Acuerdos (1804–1810), Juntas of Sept. 25, Oct. 1, 1807.

75. *Ordenanzas* (1787), Parte Tercera, Sec. I, Chap. IV. The Libros de Matrículas contain the annual results.

76. AFM, Libro de Representaciones, Ordenes, etc., Real ordenes, Oct. 19, 1794; Jan. 29, 1795; AHN, Universidades (Medicina-Serie Antigua), Leg. 1175, Parte I, Expediente of José Cristobal Abades.

77. AUC, Libro de órdenes y oficios comunicados por la Real Junta Superior Gobernativa de Cirugía al Real Colegio de San Carlos (hereinafter cited as Libro de Ordenes), Oficios of Nov. 3, Dec. 22, 1807; Libro de Acuerdos (1804–1810), Juntas of Sept. 19, Nov. 28, 1805.

Who were the young men who enrolled in San Carlos? With typical thoroughness the secretary carefully preserved the testimonies of the student's "purity of blood," the verifications of his previous education, and the courses he completed at San Carlos. Unfortunately for the historian, the documents supporting a future student's application were, at the same time, too detailed and too limited in their value. A typical applicant submitted statements from his father, his parish priest, previous teachers, and other acquaintances. The sole purpose of these was to testify to the applicant's "purity of blood" and "good life and customs." The same phrases appear again and again, suggesting that much of the verbiage was simply pro forma. These statements appear in student dossiers as late as 1842. Occasionally, a royal order declaring the "legitimacy" and "pure blood" of the applicant replaced the lengthy testament. In other cases the Crown merely dispensed the applicant from having to provide such proof.[78]

A typical statement on "purity of blood" began by tracing the subject's ancestry back several generations. Next came an extensive list of all the things the applicant and his forebears had never been—Jews, Moors, recent converts, victims of the Inquisition. Finally the writer offered a brief statement of the applicant's character. The candidate usually appeared as an obedient, docile young man who received the sacraments frequently. The statement often concluded with a sketch of its author, particularly any titles or licenses he might hold. Most of this, of course, was simply a matter of form. Nevertheless, it is noteworthy that seldom in a candidate's credentials was there ever mention of his aptitude as a student.

In modern terms, most San Carlos students were "middle class." Perhaps as many as half of them were themselves sons of surgeons or physicians. After 1800 a fair number of physicians sent their sons to San Carlos rather than to a university—convincing testimony to the growing prestige of the school. Other students came from families of civil servants or craftsmen. Occasionally the son of a laborer came to San Carlos, but this was uncommon. Whether San Carlos attracted students who would not otherwise have become surgeons is impossible to know.

The majority of students were between the ages of sixteen and

78. AHN, Universidades (Medicina–Serie Antigua), Legajos 1175–1260, contains the student files of San Carlos, arranged alphabetically. A typical file contains testimony supporting an application for admission, examination and licensing results, and the student's financial record. Many are incomplete. The observations that follow are based on Leg. 1175 (three parts) and Leg. 1232 (two parts).

twenty when they entered the school. Latin students had studied Latin, logic, mathematics, physics, and chemistry. Usually they had attended private schools run by religious orders. Apparently most secondary schools had a limited curriculum, for many students had attended a different school for one or two of the national sciences. Comparisons to contemporary education can be dangerous, but the typical student entering San Carlos was probably the equivalent of a high school sophomore today.

Not all students came to San Carlos directly from other schools. Some had practiced surgery for several years. Others dropped out of school for financial reasons and returned many years later. Even priests attended and graduated from San Carlos fairly frequently.[79] Apparently both surgery and public mores had so changed that a clergyman no longer looked down on the science as beneath his dignity.

Virtually every Spanish province was represented in the student body. However, about half the students came from Madrid, and the majority of the rest hailed from Castilian or Catalonian cities. On the other hand, most romance surgeons came from small villages, as might be expected.[80]

Like teachers everywhere, the San Carlos professors felt that most of the students never spent enough time at their studies. Though disciplinary cases were infrequent, the junta constantly sought means to encourage better use of free time. Annual prizes did little good. Most of the professors, including Gimbernat, believed that the basic problem was that the students did not room in the college. Instead, they had rooms all over Madrid and wandered the streets at will. The faculty felt that the students should be compelled to stay in the library, the clinic, or the practice room so they would make better academic progress "without the temptations that freedom presents."[81]

As the founders of San Carlos had dedicated themselves to improving "the state of the art of curing" throughout Spain, the story of San Carlos would not be complete without describing its contributions outside the classrooms. During the college's first twenty years its faculty was indeed a renowned one. Its members had had wide experi-

79. No special mention is made of this fact anywhere in the school records. However, junta discussions frequently take up the case of a priest or brother. See, for example, AUC, Libro de Acuerdos (1804–1810), Juntas of Oct. 25, Oct. 27, 1804; Sept. 20, 1805.

80. AUC, Libro de Matrícula de Cirujanos (1787–1817); Libro de Matrículas de Romancistas (1810—).

81. AFM, Libro de Representaciones, Ordenes, etc., Informe de Colegio de San Carlos, Dec. 6, 1794.

ence throughout Spain and had held important positions. Many had traveled and studied abroad. Most went on to assume high government administrative posts. The institution itself was known for its progressive methods and outstanding collections of books and exhibits. The very fact of its being located in Madrid, the center of Spanish life, added to its reputation. Thus, it is not surprising that both government officials and private practitioners frequently turned to San Carlos for advice in medical matters.

Probably the most valuable extra-classroom contributions occurred in weekly lectures held every Thursday afternoon before the private administrative meeting of the junta. The exercises were open to the public, and all students were obliged to attend. The routine was unique. First, either a professor of the school or an outside authority presented a paper. At its conclusion the director of the school appointed one of his colleagues to prepare a critique (*censura*). The following Thursday the chosen professor would present his criticism, after which the entire faculty would vote its approval or disapproval of the original paper. Following the vote, the speaker for that week would begin. Complete texts of both the formal presentation and the critique then went into the school archives. Though the formal criticisms and voting were reserved to professors, the students sometimes joined in the discussion, particularly when one of the patients in the clinic was under discussion, or when the subject matter was closely related to one of the courses. Apparently the contributions of students and others in the audience were valuable. On one occasion, after hearing a paper on a difficult obstetrical case, the secretary noted in the records the surprise of the faculty at the keen observations made by the audience. All lectures were given in Spanish in order to give them the widest possible publicity.

The topics of the papers covered the full range of surgical practice.[82] During the early years of San Carlos, professors usually delivered the papers. Often they discussed general themes they hoped the students would find useful. Juan de Nabas, professor of materia médica, for example, gave a lecture on the need to know the specific circumstances

82. The topic of each paper and the approval or disapproval of the critique are summarized in the Libros de Acuerdos. Many of the papers themselves are preserved in the AFM, uncatalogued but arranged chronologically. This collection is described in Alfredo Lapuente Mateos, "Juntas literarias y censuras en el Real Colegio de San Carlos," *Archivos iberoamericanos de historia de la medicina*, I (1949), 408–418.

The description of the non-classroom activities that follows holds true for the period after 1808 as well, and is also based on later school records.

surrounding a disease; all symptoms could not be treated alike. Neither could one always attribute specific problems to "a general malcondition of the humors."[83] As time went on, and the reputation of the school grew, most of the lectures were presented by outsiders, sometimes in person, sometimes in writing. Usually the paper was a detailed description of a particular case. A typical presentation would describe the patient, his illness or wound, the various symptoms, especially anything the author considered unusual, and finally the remedies the author had used. Often the procedure described was something new, or at least the author thought so. Many speakers were given to long reflections on the nature of disease or surgery in general, a habit some contemporaries believed very laudable.[84]

This idea of a surgeon's publicly presenting his accomplishments to his colleagues was not new. The Spanish press had carried such individual accounts for more than a decade. Though many of the procedures described in the press were fairly routine and intended for the average practitioner, the dedicated surgeon had been easily able to keep himself informed of the latest developments. Yet the San Carlos sessions provided something new. Now an inventive surgeon anywhere in the Spanish Empire could not only publicize his accomplishments but also receive an expert criticism of them. The rural practitioner, who lived in isolation but yet encountered every sort of medical problem, now had a place to which he could turn for advice.

Even a cursory glance at the summaries reveals much about the best and the worst of surgery at the end of the eighteenth century. Most of the lectures concerned themselves with the usual surgical problems: wounds, especially gunshot wounds, abscesses and tumors, ulcers, hernias, trephines. Many surgeons submitted accounts of operations they had attempted. If unsuccessful, they frequently asked what they had done wrong. In one case a surgeon sought the opinion of the San Carlos faculty on some new instruments he had fashioned.[85] Some correspondents were not even of the medical profession. Several sessions, for example, were spent discussing a Benedictine monk's description of how he dealt with a wound made by "an angry ox."[86]

83. AFM, Libros de Juntas Literarias, Vol. I, Feb. 12, 1789.

84. This aspect is discussed at length in *Memorial literio instructivo y curioso de la corte de Madrid*, Jan., 1790, pp. 57–60. The *Memorial literario y curioso* carried a regular section of "Observaciones chirúrgicas."

85. AFM, Libro de Acuerdos (1787–1804), Junta of June 25, 1793.

86. AUC, Libro de Acuerdos (1804–1810), Juntas of Nov. 29, Dec. 6, 1804; Feb. 28, 1805.

Many papers touched on subjects not traditionally considered to be the proper study of surgeons. Various types of fevers, once the exclusive province of medicine, came under frequent discussion. Occasionally a paper concerned a psychological problem, such as "severe melancholia" (*una manía melancolíca*).[87] A surprisingly large number of lectures were on obstetrical topics such as techniques of delivery and problems during pregnancy. In 1805 a surgeon submitted a description of a "Caesarian operation" he had successfully performed. According to his statement, the mother was in good health, though the fetus was dead. (Perhaps it would be better labeled a miscarriage.) Pedro Castelló, who had been assigned the critique, criticized both the description and the technique. The faculty voted not to recommend putting the surgeon's description in the *Gaceta* because "it was not an extraordinary case."

Sometimes the San Carlos professors were decidedly unimpressed with the boastful résumé a proud rural surgeon might submit. One surgeon in a small village near Segovia described a patient who had been suffering attacks of severe chest pains and shortage of breath for more than eight years. The surgeon first bled him, then fed him oxymel as an emetic. The next day he threw up a small piece of graphite covered with quicksilver (*arzojado lapiz*). The following week the critique simply noted the case was nothing unusual.[88] Nevertheless, the case is significant, for it points out that even the poor rural surgeon was interested in medical progress, aware of San Carlos, capable of writing detailed clinical reports, and eager to present his experiences to distant experts in Madrid.

Some of the papers and their criticisms reveal a modern scientific approach mixed with traditional folklore that characterized much medical practice. There were frequent references to "preternatural deliveries" (*parto preternatural*).[89] An army surgeon reported on a man "possessed by the tarantula" who was cured by music.[90] In 1807 the school heard a description of a Dominican nun who was extremely nervous, agitated, and frequently thrown into convulsions. Her own physicians had diagnosed it as the "danzo de San Vito." Sebastinán Aso

87. *Ibid.*, Junta of Nov. 8, 1804.

88. AFM, Libros de juntas literarias, Vol. VI, Jan. 2, 1806.

89. AFM, Libro de Acuerdos (1789–1804), Junta of July 2, 1793. Even the 1787 ordinances contained a provision for the professor of obstetrics to instruct his students in how to distinguish a *parto preternatural*.

90. AFM, Libro de Acuerdos (1787–1804), Junta of Jan. 29, 1788.

Travieso, the dissector, was assigned the critique. He agreed; it was a nervous affliction complicated by Saint Vitus's dance. The only remedy, he suggested, was a complete rest from all mental activity, and relaxation in a small town. "Remedies drawn from morality and religion . . . would more rapidly bring about a cure than those drawn from the pharmacy."[91] A case in 1818 shows another aspect of the transition through which popular practice was passing. An unnamed rural surgeon described his treatment of a dislocated lower jawbone, adding that many people in his village had believed the defect to be "the effect of having devils in the body."[92] One can safely assume that the Thursday afternoon assemblies were seldom boring.

On a more progressive note, the records of the assemblies also testify to the methodical reporting and sharp clinical eye of many practitioners. Typical was the presentation by Diego Rodríguez del Piño, the professor of anatomy, on a chest wound. He began with the man's age, background, and health, then gave the details of how he got the wound (a knife fight), the lapse of time before he received treatment, and what was done (five bleedings in forty hours). The patient made slow but steady progress for twenty-three days, during which the surgeon carefully recorded his diet, temperature, and general condition. But then the patient suddenly got a high fever and died seven days later despite efforts to stop the fever with cinchona (*quina*). The narrative concluded with a description of the autopsy, particularly the color and location of the wound in the chest. The critique was equally thorough. Ramón Saráis, professor of pathology, praised the report but complained of insufficient detail on the patient's unconsciousness in the hours preceding his death.[93]

The records of the Thursday afternoon exercises also reveal the close contact medical specialists in Spain maintained with their counterparts in America. Frequently a physician or surgeon in the New World was the author of the weekly dissertation. Practitioners in Puerto Rico, Mexico, and Guatemala seemed to carry on the most correspondence with the professors at San Carlos. Generally their reports were similar to those of Spanish doctors. In 1803 Narciso Esparragosa y Gallardo, the noted Guatemalan surgeon and savant who was instrumental in the founding of a surgical college in Guatemala City, submitted a

91. AUC, Libro de Acuerdos (1804–1810), Juntas of March 12, April 2, 1807.
92. AUC, Libro de Acuerdos (1817–1821), Junta of June 4, 1818.
93. AFM, Libros de juntas literarias, Vol. I, Nov. 4, 1790.

description of a pair of elastic forceps he had developed. The faculty labeled the invention "not useful," a judgment history would later prove incorrect.[94]

In addition to the weekly lectures, every school year opened with a formal lecture by one of the professors. Some of the inaugural lectures gave the professor a chance to publicize his own research. Others were of a more reflective nature, analyzing the obligations of surgery and surgical education to society at large. Sometimes a speaker used the opportunity to publicize the advanced state of his science, or to argue for the unification of surgery with medicine. Others spoke of general medical needs, such as José Ribes's lecture on the need for greater cleanliness in hospital wards.[95] Every lecture was preserved in the archives. Many were well publicized in the press.

Several San Carlos professors also wrote Spanish-language texts to further facilitate surgical education. Most widely used was the *Curso completo de anatomía* by Jaime Bonells and Ignacio Lacaba. The new statutes of 1804 instructed every professor to draw up his own course. Many of the professors were slow to put their notes together in a formal treatise, but by 1820 the school possessed some half-dozen treatises in manuscript form applicable for classroom use. Most were the work of José Rivas y Mayor, a versatile teacher who taught virtually every course during his long career.[96] Undoubtedly the most famous author to serve on the San Carlos faculty was the medical historian Antonio Hernández Morejón, who taught there during the 1820s.

The Thursday assemblies, the inaugural lectures, and the publications enabled private practitioners to benefit from the knowledge of the faculty. As time went on, official government agencies also turned to the distinguished faculty of San Carlos for advice and forced official obligations upon it. The college even assumed some of the duties traditionally performed by the Protomedicato.

From the beginning, the Crown frequently called upon Antonio Gimbernat for advice on matters unrelated to San Carlos. Apparently Gimbernat's approval was sufficient for the Hospital de Santiago in Toledo to obtain royal permission to set up a special clinic for venereal

94. AFM, Libro de Acuerdos (1787–1804), Juntas of Feb. 17, March 3, March 17, 1803. On Esparragosa, see John Tate Lanning, *The Eighteenth-Century Enlightenment in the University of San Carlos de Guatemala* (Ithaca, N.Y., 1956), pp. 276–281, 296–298.

95. AUC, Libro de Acuerdos (1804–1810), Junta of Oct. 5, 1804.

96. *Ordenanzas Generales* (1804), Cap. V; AUC, Libro de Ordenes, Oficio of Nov. 11, 1805. The manuscripts are in AFM.

diseases.[97] In 1789 the Crown requested Gimbernat's advice on reform proposals for the Barcelona college. Gimbernat eventually became the principal author of new ordinances for the school.

Confidence in Antonio Gimbernat quickly led to confidence in the school itself. A year after it opened, the faculty received an order from the Council requesting a critique of an anatomical and surgical dictionary. Two months later the college replied that the work was "incomplete, of little value, and quite possibly dangerous." After listing several errors the report concluded that the book did not merit public circulation.[98] Thus began the role of San Carlos as principal censor of medical books.

No book could be published legally in eighteenth-century Spain without a royal license. Political and religious censorship is well known, but the Crown was also concerned that only reliable scientific texts freely circulate, and that the public not be confused by "useless works." The Council of Castile, which had final authority to grant or withhold a license, frequently sought expert advice when faced with a work of science. The frequency with which San Carlos was ordered to evaluate new medical books suggests that the Council relied almost completely upon the professors there. In 1795 the statutes contained a provision whereby no book touching on surgery could be published in Spain without the approval of the Supreme Governing Board of Surgery. And the board, in turn, usually continued to forward books to the professors of San Carlos.

These men took their role as censors very seriously.[99] Usually one professor was assigned to write the critique. The entire junta of the school would then discuss it and finally vote on it, usually accepting the original judgment. From the beginning the junta chose not to state merely its approval or disapproval of a book. Instead, it submitted a detailed commentary, noting its good and bad points. The critiques frequently mentioned a book's prospects as a textbook. The job also called for linguistic skills, for the professors had both to read foreign works and evaluate their translation into Spanish. Though political censorship was strict during the years following the French Revolution,

97. *Gaceta de Madrid*, Feb. 1, 1788.

98. AFM, Libro de Representaciones, Ordenes, etc., Orden del Consejo, Oct. 4, 1788; Informe del Colegio de San Carlos, Jan. 30, 1789. The work in question was Esteban Hurtado de Mendoza, *Dictionario de anatomía y cirugía*.

99. Critiques prior to 1804 are contained verbatim in AFM, Libro de Representaciones, Ordenes, etc. Critiques after 1804 are summarized in the AUC, Libros de Acuerdos.

medical texts apparently had no trouble entering Spain. And during the reign of Charles IV the San Carlos censors never strayed from medical matters, leaving questions of politics and morality to others.

Typical was the case of a book entitled *Curso de Cirugía* by Lorenzo Nannoni, an Italian, and its translation into Spanish by Antonio Alcoriza. Two professors were assigned to evaluate it. They decided that the original work was "not a model that ought to be imitated." Its organization was confusing, and some of its practical advice was erroneous. The translator did a commendable job except for certain technical terms.[100]

Traditionally the Royal Protomedicato had been responsible for guarding the public health, but during the reign of Charles IV the government began to turn more and more to San Carlos on a variety of other matters. Censoring books was only one of its functions in its new role as medical adviser to the government. The Council asked its opinion of proposed reforms of the laws governing pharmacies.[101] On several occasions it answered requests to evaluate new treatments or new drugs. Hospitals, too, requested its opinion on new methods of treatment. Sometimes local governments asked the college to recommend a capable surgeon. In other cases the Crown requested information on "the theoretical and practical knowledge, the ability, and the character" of applicants for high medical posts.

Even the Council of the Indies called on the experts of the College of San Carlos. As part of its customary concern for public health in the New World, the Council decided to print instructions for performing Caesarian operations. In 1803 it asked the college to draw up "clear, succinct, and methodical" instructions for performing the operation. They should describe the safest methods and be clear enough for a layman to understand. The college complied. A year later the Crown issued a cédula ordering all surgeons to perform the operation according to these instructions, which were included in the printed decree. Where there was no surgeon, the parish priest was to appoint the most skilled individual available to carry out the Caesarean, again following the instructions written by San Carlos.[102]

Another aspect of government consultation with the San Carlos faculty involved the infant science of legal medicine. The most fre-

100. AFM, Libro de Representaciones, Ordenes, etc., Real orden, Aug. 15, 1795; Repuesta y censura, Oct. 16, 1795.

101. AUC, Libro de Acuerdos (1804–1810), Junta of March 9, 1808.

102. Archivo General de Indias, Gobierno, Leg. 1551, Ramo 1, Real cédula, Aranjuez, April 13, 1804; AFM, Libro de Acuerdos (1787–1805), Junta of March 3, 1803.

quent type of case concerned the question of whether a wound received in a fight was mortal in itself, or whether the victim died as a result of poor medical care. Often, of course, the college had to reply that it had insufficient information. Other questions had to do with whether a death was due to incompetence on the part of the attending physician or surgeon. One case brought by a town government in Navarre concerned the legitimacy of a baby. It seemed that the child was born five months after the wedding and the local authorities were unsure how to classify the child.[103] The legal questions were rare in the years before the Napoleonic invasion but became very common during the 1820s.

Given the public service role of the San Carlos faculty, it was natural that the Crown frequently provided funds for individual professors to study abroad. Usually the professor would take his petition for the sabbatical to the junta, which, in turn, would petition higher authorities. Rarely were the requests denied. England, France, and Italy were frequent destinations; international politics seldom intervened. The Crown usually provided travel expenses in addition to continuing the professor's normal salary. Occasionally a particularly talented student would also receive a travel grant. In 1806 the Crown even ordered the school to nominate three students for foreign study at royal expense.[104] After 1808 there are few references to such foreign study.

The public contributions of San Carlos, however, entailed more than the high qualifications of its professors. The exhibits, collections of instruments, and the library were also intended to benefit the public at large. Indeed, during its early decades the school frequently allowed private surgeons to use its facilities, when vacant, to teach their apprentices without charge.[105]

San Carlos was justifiably proud of its anatomical collection, which consisted of wax models and pieces of cadavers. In 1807 a professor at the University of Bologna offered to come to Madrid and set up an anatomical exhibit similar to the celebrated one in Berlin. The Crown asked the San Carlos faculty what it thought of the offer. The faculty answered that a foreign expert was unnecessary since the school had

103. AUC, Libro de Acuerdos (1823–1827), Junta of June 8, 1826. For other examples, see Libro de Acuerdos (1804–1810), Juntas of April 4, Aug. 18, 1804; Libro de Ordenes, Oficio of April 15, 1830.

104. AUC, Libro de Acuerdos (1804–1810), Junta of March 6, 1806. For additional examples, see the Junta of Aug. 18, 1804; AFM, Libro de Representaciones, Ordenes, etc., Informe del Colegio de San Carlos, Dec. 6, 1794; Real orden, April 18, 1804.

105. AUC, Libro de Ordenes, Oficio of Sept. 3, 1804.

excellent craftsmen of its own. San Carlos, added the junta, would have an exhibit equal to that in Berlin if it had the same money and advantageous location.[106]

Antonio Gimbernat also strove to build a collection of surgical instruments. In early 1789 the king considered giving San Carlos an outstanding collection left behind by one of his former surgeons. Unfortunately for the school, the king changed his mind and decided to keep them in the palace. Gimbernat tried another tack. After long negotiations, he devised a plan whereby the crown would loan Tomás Maseras, a master cutler, thirty thousand reales to set up a shop and make instruments. The Crown agreed, and the college gradually accumulated an exceptional collection during the next decade. By 1804 it was "complete." Two years later San Carlos apparently had more than it needed, for it offered to supply instruments to the newer colleges in Burgos and Santiago.[107]

The College of San Carlos also had a library to serve both its own students and the general public. As Gimbernat first envisioned it, it would contain books on "surgery, medicine, human and animal anatomy and related natural sciences."[108] It would be open to the public daily in the morning and afternoon. No books would circulate outside the library itself.

Building up a library was a slow undertaking. In most years little more than five hundred reales could be spent on books. Spanish ambassadors bought what they could abroad and sent them to the school, but even then customs officials had to be paid to handle them. Gimbernat was particularly interested in acquiring foreign and domestic periodicals. He turned down several opportunities to buy entire libraries so that he might use his limited resources more selectively. The library grew much faster after 1799. All Spanish authors of medical books had to send a copy to San Carlos. Government financial support increased dramatically. The Crown transferred medical collections from other libraries to San Carlos. Thus, by 1808 the library of San Carlos probably had one of the most complete medical collections in Spain.[109]

106. AUC, Libro de Acuerdos (1804–1810), Juntas of Jan. 22, Jan. 29, 1807.

107. AFM, Libro de Representaciones, Ordenes, etc., Reales ordenes, March 4, April 17, Oct. 20, 1789; Sept. 18, 1804; AUC, Libro de Acuerdos (1810–1816), Junta of Nov. 29, 1816.

108. *Ordenanzas* (1787), Parte Quinta, Sec. I, Cap. I.

109. AFM, Libro de Cuentas (1786–1815); Libro de Representaciones, Ordenes, etc., Reales ordenes, Nov. 24, Dec. 29, 1789; Joaquín Malo y Calvo, *Reseña histórica de la Biblioteca de la Facultad de Medicina de Madrid* (Madrid, 1875), pp. 12–24. The

Despite these myriad activities, the basic function of the College of San Carlos was always that of training surgeons. San Carlos made the latest medical knowledge and techniques available to young Spaniards. Its graduates were as well educated as any in Europe. The curriculum they studied was more advanced than university education anywhere. The emphasis on research exposed them to the exciting search for new knowledge; now Spaniards were no longer merely following in the footsteps of foreigners. In many respects San Carlos had also assumed many of the traditional responsibilities of the university and the Royal Protomedicato. The college admirably combined teaching and public service. This was as it should be, for both were essential to "restoring surgery to its proper position."[110]

---

library was the beginning of the present library of the Facultad de Medicina of the University of Madrid.

110. Gimbernat, *Oración inaugural* (1768).

CHAPTER VI

# SAN CARLOS AND MEDICAL REFORM UNDER CHARLES IV

WHEN CHARLES IV came to the throne in 1788 the proponents of Enlightenment and reform had won many victories, particularly in education. University courses now followed modern texts. New schools untied to the old traditions offered instruction in the "useful arts." Powerful guilds such as those of university professors, physicians, and surgeons had lost much of their traditional autonomy. The Crown influenced educational affairs as never before. The unspoken alliance between Spanish liberals and the Crown had brought about reform and centralization together.

Reformers such as Antonio Gimbernat were not content to rest on the success of a few institutions, however. No one in 1788 claimed the work of reform was complete. Not only was there a great deal more to accomplish, but the forces of tradition were still numerous and vocal. As a result, the next two decades consisted of efforts to extend the fruits of reform throughout Spain and to suppress outmoded ideas and institutions once and for all.

From its inception the surgeons of San Carlos had expected that their college would become the standard for surgical education everywhere. Almost immediately they endeavored to impose the progressive features of San Carlos on surgical colleges throughout the country and to encourage the establishment of additional colleges that duplicated the school in Madrid. The individual innovation that characterized the first three colleges was no longer to be. Surgical colleges, like universities, were to conform to national standards.

By the 1790s, however, the reforming surgeons realized that the reform of surgery, indeed, of the entire medical profession, could not be successful as long as the colleges of surgery existed in a vacuum. Romance surgery had to be suppressed or brought under the supervision of the colleges. Even medicine was not immune from the efforts of the reformers. During the 1790s San Carlos became the model for further university reform and the creation of obligatory clinical training for physicians. As the decade drew to a close, Gimbernat seemed close to realizing his ultimate dream: the unification of medicine and surgery under the progressive leadership of men such as himself.

As in the past, the reformers needed the continued support of the Crown and a consensus among themselves in order to be effective. Unfortunately, neither of these occurred. Although Charles IV adhered to his predecessor's objectives of reform, royal control, and standardization, both the French Revolution and the personality of Manuel Godoy caused serious divisions among the reformers and created an unbridgeable chasm between progressive Spaniards and the Crown. So great was the rupture that enlightened Spaniards found themselves on opposing sides during the civil war that followed the invasion by Napoleon.

The French Revolution itself posed serious questions for the Spanish reformers who for generations had looked to France as a model.[1] The Revolution stood for change on a grand scale, but it also challenged much that all Spaniards held sacred. Even most Jansenists could not easily dismiss its threat to religion, and few reformers were prepared to challenge legitimate political authority. Indeed, the success of Spanish intellectuals was a direct result of the growing absolutism of the Crown. They knew that the Spanish monarchy was probably more progressive than were many Spanish subjects.

Until 1792 Charles IV relied on the enlightened ministers who had served his predecessor, the Conde de Floridablanca and the Conde de Aranda. Floridablanca drew back at the excesses of the French Revolution, however, and imposed rigid censorship. Aranda, who remained an admirer of France, became discredited as the Revolution turned to the left and Jacobin propaganda poured into Spain. Finally, Charles dismissed them both and appointed Manuel Godoy as First Minister.

Manuel Godoy, one of the most perplexing men in Spanish history, dominated Spain from 1792 until 1808. According to one historian, his

1. The following description of the reign of Charles IV is based on Hans Roger Madol, *Godoy, el primer dictador de nuestro tiempo*, trans. G. Sans Huelin and M. Sandmann (Madrid, 1966); Jacques Chastenet, *Godoy, Master of Spain, 1792–1808*, trans. J. F. Huntington (London, 1953); Herr, *The Eighteenth Century Revolution*, pp. 240–434; Gabriel H. Lovett, *Napoleon and the Birth of Modern Spain* (2 vols.; New York, 1965), I, 12–24; Manuel Godoy, *Memorias críticas y apologéticas* (2 vols.; "Biblioteca de Autores Españoles," vols. 88–89), esp. I, 193–223; Carlos Seco Serrano, "Godoy: El hombre y el político," in Godoy, *Memorias*, I, vii–cxxxviii; Segundo Serrano Poncela, "Godoy y los ilustrados," in *Formas de vida hispánica* (Madrid, 1963), pp. 126–136; Raymond Carr, *Spain, 1808–1939* (Oxford, 1966), pp. 43–83.

power was more absolute than that of any subsequent ruler before Generalissimo Francisco Franco.[2] He was an easy man to hate. Suspected of being the queen's lover, he had risen from an insignificant post in the Royal Guards to First Minister of the king in only a few years. He was vain, ambitious, and crude. He set out to complete the work of reform and assured himself he could do it singlehandedly. Yet the man was not incompetent. For thirteen years he managed to keep Napoleon out of Spain. His policy lacked nobility but not pragmatism. In a sense he attempted to deal with Napoleon as he dealt with Charles IV. In 1808, though, he discovered to his dismay that one could not so easily outdo Napoleon in craftiness.

Godoy continued his predecessors' policy of supporting royal institutions dedicated to science and culture at the expense of the universities. He readily provided funds for scientific and cultural pursuits, and tried to foment a spirit of progress as well. Under his aegis were founded the Royal School of Practical Medicine, the School of Veterinary Medicine, the Corps of Cosmographical Engineers, and the Madrid Astronomical Observatory, to name a few. Government support of existing institutions and programs continued unabated both in Spain and America. At the same time he had no patience for the universities, whatever the merit of their position. By the 1790s, paradoxically, the universities not only continued to represent reaction and obscurantism but at the same time were looked upon as hotbeds of radicalism sympathetic to the French Revolution. Thus, under Godoy, reform and standardization were to continue, but on his terms. The caution and dialogue that had characterized educational reform under Charles III all but ceased to exist.[3]

Despite Godoy's progressive accomplishments and his own intense desire to be accepted as an enlightened reformer, the First Secretary had little success in winning the unqualified praise and support of liberal intellectuals. Many simply refused to accept a young upstart who appeared to have achieved power through means that were irregular, to say the least. Others believed that Godoy lacked the competence to continue the policies of Charles III. As a result, the reforms of Godoy were much more sporadic, much less planned, than those of earlier

2. Carr, *Spain*, p. 82.

3. For medical reforms under Godoy, see García del Real, *Medicina en España*, pp. 488–499. For reforms in higher education, see Antonio Alvarez de Morales, *La "Ilustración" y la reforma de la universidad en la España del siglo XVIII* (Madrid, 1971), pp. 159–201.

reigns. The ministers of Charles III had acted perhaps too carefully in seeking advice from every quarter and planning for every contingency. Under Godoy radical change seemed to spring up overnight, creating as much confusion as progress. Both his own personality and his lack of support from intellectuals seem to have been responsible for the situation.

It is risky, however, to characterize all intellectuals as being of one mind. Some liberals bitterly opposed the regime,[4] but others, realizing that they were still a minority in Spanish society, recognized that Godoy was sympathetic to their aims. They were willing to work with him in spite of their personal opinions. This pliability was particularly true of the directors of those institutions usually associated with the Enlightenment. Eugenio Izquierdo, for example, the director of the Museum of Natural History, undertook several diplomatic missions for Godoy. Antonio Gimbernat was also typical of this pragmatic approach. Completely committed to the betterment of surgical education, he was willing to cooperate with anyone who gave him support. And so, gradually, a small coterie of intellectuals, many of them French sympathizers, gathered around Godoy.

In 1797 Godoy initiated a succession of ministerial changes that culminated in one of the most liberal governments Spain had ever seen. Not known for their caution and tact, these young ministers exhibited little sympathy for any traditional institution, including the universities. By mid-1798, Mariano Luis de Urquijo, a brash young man who had no patience for the opinions of those he did not respect, had replaced Godoy as First Minister. The new secretary of grace and justice, who had responsibility for internal affairs, was José Antonio Caballero. Caballero was convinced that both the universities and the professions were hopelessly decadent and should be replaced.

As we shall see, these rapid changes in government would provide the surgeons of San Carlos with the opportunity to fulfill their wildest dreams. If university medicine and the Protomedicato were less progressive than San Carlos, why not let the colleges of surgery assume their functions? Caballero would agree.

The liberal regime was short-lived, however. Events in France and the increasingly intense conflict between Jansenists and ultramontanes in Spain, a conflict that predated Charles III, brought the Urquijo government down in 1800. The liberals had attempted too much too

4. Herr, *The Eighteenth Century Revolution*, pp. 324 ff., emphasizes this faction.

fast and had underestimated the opposition. Godoy regained his former influence, considerably chastened and more conservative. His cousin, Pedro Ceballos, a leading conservative, became First Minister.

The second eight years of Godoy differed little from the first, except that the façade of ultra-liberalism was missing. Angered by the lack of appreciation liberals had given him, Godoy now chose to follow a middle-of-the-road policy. To be sure, his pro-French foreign policy continued and was partly responsible for later conspiracies against Charles IV. But domestic policies became more moderate. Godoy undid the radical reforms of the Urquijo ministry and made few innovations. Reformers such as Antonio Gimbernat lost their traditional influence at court. Now Godoy not only listened to conservative interests but often followed their advice. Of course, Godoy still supported reform and patronized the arts and sciences. He was no reactionary, but he was a man who was dedicated to his own future above all else. And that future was no longer tied to the most liberal reformers of Spain. By 1808 few mourned his fall from power. He remained an ardent reformer only in the eyes of the anti-French supporters of the reactionary Ferdinand VII.[5]

Thus, Manuel Godoy was a mixed blessing for Spanish reform. During his years of power progressive institutions flourished and the spirit of reform remained. The histories of individual schools such as San Carlos reveal no break with the past upon his rise to power. Indeed, his propensity for rapid decisions often made innovation easier to bring about. On the other hand, one detects a decline in the morale of those intellectuals who had originated most of the ideas of change. Under Godoy the growing centralization of power reached the point where those in high positions hardly seemed to listen to advice from below. Moreover, the very concept of reform from above became discredited. The popular disgust that surrounded the Godoy government caused many Spaniards to cease looking to an alliance between intellectuals and a centralized monarchy as the most desirable method of bringing about change.

Antonio Gimbernat exhibited little interest in the vagaries of ministerial politics. Always more concerned with the practical problems of reform than the ideologies or personalities behind them, he was willing to cooperate with any government that would further the prog-

5. Ironically, Godoy looked back on his years in power as a time of great reform. His *Memorias* devote countless pages to recounting his progressive accomplishments, giving the impression that he ruled a nation of intense intellectual activity.

ress of surgery. Between 1788 and 1808 Gimbernat used every available opportunity to impose his ideas beyond the College of San Carlos itself.

His first opportunity arose in 1789 when several controversies regarding seniority at the Barcelona college opened the door to revising the whole curriculum there. When word of the dispute reached Madrid, the Crown sent the report to Custodio Gutiérrez for advice. Gimbernat and his colleagues used the opportunity to write a general critique of the Barcelona school. They advocated assigning a specific subject to each professor, stricter entrance requirements, and extending the course from four to five years.[6]

The efforts of San Carlos to remake other schools in its own image proved successful. In 1790 the Barcelona faculty began work on revising the statutes there. Four years later the Crown, impressed with Gimbernat's criticisms and with his accomplishments at San Carlos, named him director of the Barcelona school.[7] Although Gimbernat did not assume supervision of the school's day-to-day operation, the new position enabled him to influence the new statutes.

In 1795 the quest for uniformity culminated with the creation of a Superior Board of Surgical Colleges (*Junta Superior Gubernativa de los Reales Colegios de Cirugía*).[8] Citing "the continual discord among the personnel of the Royal Colleges of Surgery," the royal decree entrusted the new body with sole responsibility for supervising the schools. Gimbernat and two other San Carlos professors were named to the board, establishing the precedent whereby San Carlos professors would continue to serve on the supervisory body. Two months later the Crown approved the new statutes for Barcelona, which included some improvements upon those of San Carlos, and imposed them on the Madrid school as well.

The San Carlos professors were initially angered by these developments. The faculty itself, not outside administrative bodies, should revise the curriculum, they argued. The school was losing control of its own destiny. It was subject to the whims of higher authorities in matters the faculty itself was most qualified to judge.[9]

In fact, however, these developments imposed the principles of San Carlos on every other school of surgery. The new statutes essentially

6. AFM, Libro de Representaciones, Ordenes, etc., Real orden, Feb. 6, 1789; Informe del Colegio de San Carlos, May 15, 1789.

7. AGS, Secretaría de Hacienda, Leg. 949, Expediente del Colegio de Barcelona, materias diversas, Real aviso, March 3, 1794.

8. AFM, Libro de Representaciones, Ordenes, etc., Real orden, April 19, 1795.

9. *Ibid.*, Representación del Colegio de San Carlos, Nov. 12, 1795.

preserved the order of courses, the matriculation requirements, and the specialization of instructors. Moreover, former San Carlos professors dominated the Superior Board. Thus, although San Carlos as an institution became subordinate to another body, the principles of its founders dominated surgical education throughout Spain. In effect, San Carlos had become the model for colleges of surgery everywhere.

The preeminence of San Carlos soon became more apparent. The Barcelona statutes were imposed on the Cádiz school in 1796, and the Superior Board replaced the naval authorities in providing direct supervision.[10] When the Crown created additional colleges, they, too, conformed to Gimbernat's statutes. Even American surgical education eventually conformed to that of San Carlos. For example, a new college of surgery in Guatemala, authorized by the Crown in 1804, was to follow the statutes of San Carlos.[11]

In addition to improving the colleges themselves, Gimbernat had long been concerned about the prevalence of uneducated, untrained romance surgeons. As long as the romance surgeon still dominated the profession, the educated San Carlos graduate would have little influence. As early as 1794 Gimbernat urged that at least a few years' study at a surgical school should be mandatory for all practitioners.[12] His continued influence on the Superior Board was probably responsible for the 1797 cédula providing that all romance surgeons in the Madrid area had to attend San Carlos for three years. Potential romance surgeons elsewhere would have to serve three years as hospital interns. Private instructors could no longer offer lessons on their own.[13] Now romance surgeons as well were to acquire the academic credentials that would accord them the status of a profession rather than a trade. At the same time the colleges of surgery had acquired a role in the licensing of all practitioners.

As the surgical colleges increased their influence and stature, the universities became victims of the most hostile government attacks yet. Godoy believed that the new scientific institutions such as San Carlos held far more promise than university reform; one of his sub-

10. *Ibid.*, Oficio de la Junta Superior, May 17, 1796.

11. Lanning, *The Eighteenth-Century Enlightenment in . . . Guatemala*, p. 296; Carlos Martínez Durán, *Las ciencias médicas en Guatemala* (3rd ed.; Guatemala City, 1964), pp. 513–516.

12. AFM, Libro de Representaciones, Ordenes, etc., Informe del Colegio de San Carlos, Dec. 6, 1794.

13. AHN, Consejos, Leg. 1845, Exp. 10, Real cédula . . . en que se prescribe el Método que ha de observarse en el Tribunal de Proto-Cirujanato en los exámenes de Cirujanos . . . , May 12, 1797.

ordinates, the Conde de Cabarrús, even toyed with the idea of suppressing the universities entirely.[14] Although Godoy himself never went that far, he was disinclined to give university faculties any hearing, even when their ideas had merit. As a result, even though liberal professors continued to propose further revisions, government ministers and their appointed committees actually drew up the reforms. The faculty of San Carlos, with its close ties in government, had considerably more influence at court than any university faculty. Thus, the insignificant role played by the universities in educational reform during the reign of Charles IV cannot be blamed completely on the conservatism of their faculties; rather it was because Godoy completely ignored the efforts of liberals within the universities to initiate their own reforms.

In the field of medicine the dominant position of the Madrid reformers was particularly crucial. Godoy was determined to bring uniformity and royal control to the entire medical profession. University medicine was just one aspect of a broader concern. The very reformers who had broken away from university medicine were now writing the rules for the entire profession. As a result, the principal innovation in the training of physicians did not even occur within the faculties of medicine.

By 1790, of course, the universities were no longer the decadent institutions of earlier decades. Indeed, Salamancan graduates of the 1790s became the liberals who dominated the Cortes in 1810.[15] Faculties of medicine offered a curriculum that included modern texts, an emphasis on anatomy, stricter degree standards, and a logical progression of courses.[16] Yet even the most progressive university faculty appeared backward in comparison with San Carlos. Other problems contributed further to the universities' reactionary image. Insufficient funds, vacant chairs, and a scarcity of students continued to retard their development. Individual professors remained hostile to change. The pace of reform varied greatly from place to place. Valencia and Seville, which participated in the growth of regional universities at the expense of the three "national" ones, were particularly progressive. Two of the traditionally

14. Alvarez de Morales, *La "Ilustración,"* p. 169.

15. See Juan Marichal, "From Pistoica to Cádiz: A Generation's Itinerary, 1786–1812," in A. Owen Aldridge (ed.), *The Ibero-American Enlightenment* (Urbana, Ill., 1971), pp. 100–101.

16. AHN, Consejos, Leg. 5444, Exp. 1, Expediente formado . . . para que las Universidades del Reyno informasen por que autores se enseñan todas las Facultades . . . , 1796.

prestigious institutions, Salamanca and Alcalá, however, provide contrasting examples of the success of university reform in medicine.

The faculty of medicine at Salamanca remained progressive, innovative, and eager to adopt the latest reforms. In 1789, after reviewing the experience of the preceding eighteen years, it drew up a new plan of studies that incorporated many of the features of San Carlos.[17] Its progressive proposals included a mandatory background in the natural sciences, courses in botany, materia médica, and surgery for all students, a clinic, and courses based on subject matter instead of authors. Unfortunately, the university cloister did not approve the plan, and no further action was taken.

At the University of Alcalá, however, conditions were quite different. Between 1789 and 1795 only eight students received medical degrees, compared with 68 in theology and 336 in canons. For several years, two of the four chairs in medicine were vacant.[18] Moreover, some of the Alcalá faculty even doubted the wisdom of the reforms already in effect. The university, for example, failed to acquire a competent anatomist because it could not pay an adequate salary. In 1795, rather than attempt to raise the pay for the position, two medical professors petitioned the Crown for permission to suspend classes in the subject. The medical classes contained enough anatomy for a physician, they argued; an entire course in anatomy was "superficial and useless, if not actually harmful," considering the time it consumed. A certain amount of greed may have reinforced the petitioners' traditional thinking, for they also suggested that the salary for the chair of anatomy be divided among the rest of the faculty.[19] Although the Crown turned down the request, such thinking did little to instill confidence in the future of the universities.

Tradition was particularly potent in the formal ceremonies for advanced degrees. The licentiate and doctorate were purely honorary in Spanish education and did not signify advanced study or research.

17. AHN, Consejos, Leg. 5467, Exp. 23, Plan de Enseñanza de Medicina de la Universidad de Salamanca, 1789; Addy, *The Enlightenment in . . . Salamanca*, pp. 175–177. There is no direct evidence of communication between the reformers at Salamanca and those at San Carlos, though it seems likely each was aware of the other's activities.

18. AHN, Consejos, Libro 2711, Libro de Matrículas de Universidades (essentially a catalogue of expedientes on faculty vacancies and oposiciones); Leg. 5436, Exp. 14, 1794, contains tables of statistics for all universities.

19. AHN, Consejos, Leg. 5436, Exp. 25, Los Catedráticos de Instituciones Médicas de la Universidad de Alcalá sobre que continue la suspensión de la . . . Cátedra de Anatomía . . . , 1795.

To receive such a degree, one had only to pay a fee and deliver a formal lecture before the university faculty. Since government reformers had largely ignored the advanced degrees, the faculty at Alcalá was able to continue the traditional practices in spite of the reforms. As a result, the candidate who had studied Boerhaave during his collegiate year was obliged to give a lecture on a point from the classical authors in order to win the prestigious higher degrees.[20]

Nevertheless, by 1790, the principal shortcoming in the training of physicians lay not in the classroom but in the lack of any clinical experience outside it. The university graduate, though familiar with the latest medical theory, had no practical experience. Most likely he had completed four years of medical studies without ever coming in contact with a patient. The traditional requirement of two years of practice with a licensed physician proved equally ineffective; all too often the two years of practice amounted to little more than two years of semiservitude. The only exception was the ever-progressive University of Valencia, which had initiated clinical training in 1786.

During the 1790s the government of Godoy took several important steps to remedy this unhappy situation. The government was little inclined to turn to the universities, apparently in the belief that what the universities neglected was better entrusted to new institutions under tight royal control. Accordingly, in 1795 the Crown created the Royal School of Practical Medicine (*Estudio Real de Medicina Práctica*) to provide physicians with formal clinical training. Two years later its two-year course became mandatory for all future physicians in Castile. Just as university neglect of surgery had led to royal colleges of surgery, so, too, university neglect of clinical training led to royal schools of clinical training.

Not all university physicians, of course, had been unaware of the need for clinical practice. The Salamancan medical faculty had included a chair of clinical training in its reform proposals of 1789. The University of Valencia already had one. Even the Protomedicato recognized the value of formal hospital clinical training.[21]

By the 1790s special clinics unaffiliated with universities also existed in France and England, where faculties of medicine appeared even less open to innovation. In Spain the initiative for special clinical training

20. AHN, Consejos, Leg. 5436, Exp. 13, Representación de Joseph Penilla, Dec. 30, 1793.

21. AHN, Consejos, Leg. 5444, Exp. 1, Informe de la Universidad de Valencia, 1796; Iborra, "Memoria," pp. 292–293.

came from the medical advisers at court. There appears to have been no prior consultation with the universities. San Carlos apparently provided the model.[22] The school itself was located in the new section of the Hospital General of Madrid next to the San Carlos clinic. Thus, San Carlos not only introduced clinical training to surgery but made it an essential part of medical training as well.

The statutes of the Royal School of Practical Medicine closely followed the principles set down by Antonio Gimbernat for San Carlos.[23] The vigorous oposición, the formal inaugural lectures, the careful observations of the patients, the making of rounds by a professor followed by his students were all similar. The course lasted two years and was open only to university graduates. There were two chairs, "chronic diseases" and "acute diseases." Each professor supervised a clinic of twelve patients, carefully chosen to illustrate his lectures. The course consisted of lectures, periodic examinations, and work in the clinic. After completing the two-year course, the bachelor of medicine was eligible for a physician's license. Thus, in essence, the school offered future physicians the same day-to-day practical experience that had been available to surgeons for several years.

Two years after founding the school, the Crown began to take steps to make the Madrid school the model for clinical training everywhere, and to make such training compulsory for all future physicians. New statutes for the University of Valencia, approved in August 1797, clearly declared that the clinic there was to pattern itself after the one in Madrid.[24] Even American medicine followed the Madrid model. In Mexico, Viceroy Branciforte, having heard of the Madrid clinic, initiated plans to establish a similar institution there. The Crown established a Mexican clinic in 1804 and made attendance compulsory four years later.[25]

22. A later proposal for a similar clinical school at Salamanca explicitly states that the Royal School of Practical Medicine was established as a result of the success of the San Carlos clinic. (AHN, Consejos, Leg. 5468, Parte 1, Exp. 58, Plan de Estudios de la Facultad Médica, 1804.)

23. ARP, Leg. 691, *Ordenanzas que S.M. manda observar por la enseñanza de Medicina Práctica en las Cátedras nuevamente establecidas en el Hospital General de Madrid, con la denominación de Estudio Real de Medicina práctica* (Madrid, 1795), Nov. 23, 1795 (hereinafter cited as *Ordenanzas de Medicina Práctica* [1795].) The description of the school that follows is based on these ordinances. I have not located any documents describing the origin of the school.

24. AHN, Consejos, Leg. 5444, Exp. 14, Parte 1, *Ordenanzas para el gobierno de la Cátedra de Medicina Práctica establecida por S.M. en la Universidad de Valencia* (Madrid, 1797), Aug. 30, 1797.

25. Francisco Fernández del Castillo, *La Facultad de Medicina según el Archivo de la Real y Pontificia Universidad de México* (Mexico City, 1953), pp. 265–275, contains the relevant documents.

In October 1797 the Crown went a step further, declaring that after 1799 all future physicians would have to study "practical medicine" for two years before obtaining a license.[26] Since only the University of Valencia offered such instruction, all other university graduates would have to spend two years in Madrid. Although the universities had never supervised the years of practice, they were quick to react to this new threat to their preeminence. The full cloister at Salamanca immediately approved the medical reform plan that had been collecting dust since 1789 and petitioned Madrid to allow the university its own chair of clinical training.[27] However, its pleas went unheeded; the government had other plans for the future of medicine.

The new school also provided potential competition for San Carlos. The two schools competed for funds. The library of the surgical college suffered since the library of the new school, instead of San Carlos, now received a copy of every published medical work. Even the traditional scorn of physicians for surgeons threatened cooperation between schools. The clinical students often hurled insults at the surgical students, calling them "barbers" and "toothpullers."[28] It would take more than royal decrees and new schools to eliminate the prejudice of centuries.

The reforms also led to considerable confusion. According to law, all surgeons had to attend a college of surgery and all physicians had to attend a clinical school after getting the bachelor's degree. In practice, exemptions were easy to obtain. The ultimate regulation of the two professions was divided among universities, royal schools, and governing boards. In its effort to standardize education and licensing, the government had introduced many innovations without fully comprehending their effect on the professions as a whole. Spain had but three schools of surgery and two of clinical training that were now obligatory for all surgeons and physicians, respectively. Only the severe shortage of candidates for these professions made the requirements realistic. In 1798, only some sixty physicians and 150 surgeons received licenses in Madrid.[29] Indeed, the remarkable feature of Spanish medi-

26. The Royal Order, which I have not seen, is described in detail in AHN, Consejos, Leg. 5467, Exp. 23, Representación del claustro de la Universidad de Salamanca, Nov. 18, 1797.

27. *Ibid.*; also discussed in Addy, *The Enlightenment in . . . Salamanca*, p. 204.

28. AUC, Libro de Acuerdos (1804–1810), Junta of Feb. 5, 1807.

29. AGS, Hacienda-Dirección General del Tesoro (hereinafter cited as Dir. Gral. del Tesoro), Inventario 24, Leg. 977. This contains a list of candidates approved by the Protomedicato. The low number of physicians may mean that most candidates for that license did not study in Madrid as the law required.

cine was that these five schools could handle the needs of the entire profession.

In 1799, under the liberal Urquijo ministry, three decades of institutional reform culminated in a remarkable series of steps that radically overhauled the entire structure of medicine and surgery. In February the Crown united the Royal School of Practical Medicine and the College of San Carlos into one institution and placed it under the Superior Administrative Board of the Royal Colleges of Surgery.[30] A month later the Crown approved detailed statutes for the new school of medicine and surgery.[31] On April 20, before the school had a chance to adjust to its new condition, the Crown went a significant step further and united medicine, surgery, and pharmacy into one profession.[32] The age-old distinctions between physician and surgeon suddenly came to an end. Spain now had one profession in the practice of the healing arts. To enforce the new structure the Crown suppressed the Protomedicato and created a new General Governing Board of the United Faculty (*Junta General de Gobierno de la Facultad Reunida*). This new body consisted of the senior physicians and surgeons from the old separate bodies, although future members would have to be competent in both branches of medicine. The members were dubbed *físicos* in order to avoid any association with the former divisions of medicine.

Although specific documentary evidence tracing the decision to unify the medical profession is sparse, there is little doubt as to the men and motives behind it. As usual, unification came about as the result of the cooperation between reformers within the profession and progressive royal ministers. Three of the four authors of the regulations that established the united faculty were closely associated with San Carlos: Antonio Gimbernat, who dominated the deliberations, Pedro

30. AFM, Libro de Representaciones, Ordenes, etc., Reales órdenes, Feb. 19, Feb. 27, 1799.

31. "Artículos aprobados por S.M. en Real Orden del 12 de Marzo [1800], para la reunión de los Estudios de Medicina y Cirugiá, y establecimiento de dos nuevos Colegios de esta Facultad" (hereinafter cited as "Artículos para la reunión de los Estudios"), in *Reales órdenes expedidas en el año de 1799 por la primera Secretaría de Estado para la reunión del estudio y exercicio de la Medicina y Cirugía, y erección de una Junta General de Gobierno de esta Facultad reunida* (collection of royal orders hereinafter cited as *Ordenes para la reunión*) (Madrid, 1799). Copies of this collection exist in ARP, Leg. 689, and AHN, Universidades, Sig. 1232.

32. "Artículos aprobados por S.M. en Real Orden de 20 de Abril, para la reunión de la Medicina con la Cirugía, que deben regir provisionalmente hasta que se forme una ordenanza que abrace todas las reglas precisas para el Gobierno de esta Facultad Reunida" (hereinafter cited as "Artículos para la Facultad Reunida"), in *Ordenes para la reunión.*

Custodio Gutiérrez, and Leonardo Galli, a member of the Superior Board from Barcelona.[33] These three, plus Juan Gámez, another San Carlos professor, became físicos on the new governing board. All four held royal titles and had frequently advised the Crown in the past. The institutions they represented were themselves an innovation. As individuals, they had little patience with the demands of tradition and custom. Within the realm of medicine they played a role similar to the liberal advisers of Charles III. They were a minority, but they had the ear of key ministers. Unification achieved their longtime objective of removing the inferior status of surgery. Gimbernat, who undoubtedly engineered the enactment of unification, not only served on the general governing board but also personally drew up the new curriculum of the royal schools of medicine and surgery.[34]

Unification of the profession was only possible, of course, with government support. Mariano Luis de Urquijo, the impetuous Francophile, was not one to worry about possible protests from established interests. His secretary of grace and justice, José Antonio Caballero, was happy to support any reform that would further reduce the influence of the universities.[35]

The advocates of unification had several objectives. Reform would suppress the gradations of practitioners that had created so much bitterness and led to so many lawsuits. For Gimbernat and his colleagues, unification would dispel the lingering belief that surgery was a second-rate profession despite the new colleges and its separation from the Protomedicato. Now everyone would study the same material, graduate from the same schools, and treat the same illnesses. Unification would restore harmony to the profession. The 1795 statutes for the surgical colleges had already included internal medicine as part of the curriculum. Complete unification of education in all branches of medicine was the next logical step. Moreover, the distinction between internal and external diseases was unrealistic in the day-to-day experiences of many practitioners.

Unification also provided the opportunity to impose higher educational standards on the profession by removing medicine from the

33. Galli names the authors of the reform in an 1822 pamphlet on the same issue, *Contestacíon al informe . . . de las Décades médico-quirúrgicas y farmacéuticas, o sea juste vindicación de los autores del estudio reunido de Medicina y Cirugía* (Madrid, 1822).

34. AFM, Libro de Acuerdos para la Junta Superior, Orden de la Junta de la Facultad Reunida, Aug. 8, 1799, names Gimbernat as the author of the plan of studies.

35. On Caballero, see Alvarez de Morales, *La "Ilustración,"* p. 180.

backward universities. San Carlos undeniably provided better training than most medical faculties. Unification would provide this training for future physicians as well. It was the logical culmination of years of reforming the universities, restricting their powers, and standardizing their curricula. The royal colleges were not tied to tradition and were more easily regulated. In 1807 Gimbernat pleaded for unification once again as the only way of improving medical education. Medicine was most effectively taught in special schools.[36] Vicente Majaisla, a member of the Academy of Medicine, believed that advances in the natural sciences were doomed to failure as long as the universities dominated higher education.[37] The future of "useful education" lay in specialized schools and institutes alone.

One additional factor that probably influenced both the medical reformers and the Crown ministers was the example of France. Though its influence is impossible to measure, at least some intellectuals admired the specific reforms of the French Revolution without necessarily accepting its complete ideology. The faculty of medicine at the University of Paris, more outdated than any Spanish university, was suppressed in 1790. In 1794 the Convention established new state medical schools with a single curriculum that combined medicine and surgery.[38] An anonymous member of the Madrid Academy of Medicine prepared a paper showing how the French system might be applied in Spain. Leonardo Galli, one of the four authors of unification, quoted extensively from the French plan of studies when he attempted to justify reunification years later.[39] Unfortunately, the similarity between the united faculty and the French system later caused unification to be branded as a "liberal" arrangement.

In any event, the General Governing Board of the United Faculty, itself dominated by progressive surgeons, governed all medical education and licensing between 1799 and 1801. It was responsible for setting curriculum requirements, establishing fees, and supervising all faculty. The royal colleges, the faculties of medicine at the universities, and the military medical corps were under its direction.

The new board used its broad powers to create a system of medical-

36. Dictamen de Gimbernat, 1807, quoted in Agustín de Gimbernat, *Noticia de Gimbernat*, pp. 55–57.

37. Academia de Medicina de Madrid, Varios papeles de Estudios Médicos (1801), Letter of Vicente Majaisla to Ignacio Luzuriaga, March 18, 1801.

38. Ackerknecht, *Medicine at the Paris Hospital*, p. 32.

39. Academia de Medicina de Madrid, Varios papeles de Estudios Médicos (1801), Extracto del Proyecto de Ley sobre la instrucción pública en Francia . . . acomodado a lo que puede convenirnos en España; Galli, *Contestación al informe*, p. 87.

surgical colleges patterned after San Carlos that would have a virtual monopoly of all medical education and licensing in Spain.[40] The system would consist initially of San Carlos, the existing surgical colleges in Cádiz and Barcelona, and two new schools to be established in Burgos and Santiago. Each school would offer a single six-year curriculum that would include both internal medicine and surgery; the clinical training of the last two years would discard the traditional distinction between medical and surgical cases. The curriculum itself was essentially that of San Carlos after 1795, with additional time spent on internal diseases. Moreover, the five schools would be the only bodies in Spain that could grant licenses to practice either medicine or surgery. (Graduates of university medical faculties still had to study two years of clinical medicine in one of the five schools.) In October 1799 the general board took the final step toward unification by declaring that the medical-surgical colleges could license their graduates to practice both medicine and surgery. Thus, medicine in all its aspects was now a single profession over which the royal colleges exercised complete control.

The new regulations tremendously boosted the position of San Carlos and her sister schools at the expense of the universities. The progressive curriculum of San Carlos was now the only prerequisite for practicing medicine. A small college that had been founded to raise the level of a despised profession now led the way in medical training. The university had become separated from the professional training of future doctors; for the first time in more than three centuries a student could become a licensed physician without ever having attended a university. Perhaps the final insult to university traditions was a decree declaring that the examinations for the degree of bachelor of arts and bachelor of medicine, both of which the royal colleges also granted, were to be conducted in Spanish.[41]

Meanwhile, the merger of San Carlos and the School of Practical Medicine in Madrid proceeded smoothly. As after every change, the junta faced a flurry of petitions for exemptions to the new rules. Medical students were readily allowed, as in the old days, to use time

40. The following is based on "Artículos para la reunión de los Estudios" (March 12, 1799); AFM, Libro de Acuerdos para la Junta Superior, Ordenes de la Junta de la Facultad Reunida, April 20, May 3, June 5, June 14, Aug. 8, Oct. 31, 1799.

41. AFM, Libro de Acuerdos para la Junta Superior, Orden de la Junta de la Facultad Reunida, Jan. 9, 1800. The University of Salamanca was more fortunate than most, having successfully petitioned its alumnus, the First Secretary Urquijo, to include it among the schools of medicine and surgery. (Addy, *The Enlightenment in . . . Salamanca*, pp. 208–209.)

spent assisting private physicians in place of the two years at San Carlos.[42] Licensed San Carlos graduates demanded accreditation as physicians also, for which two additional years of service in the clinic were usually required.[43] Meanwhile, many former university students transferred to San Carlos and sought credit for the years they had completed. The decisions varied. While the student problems continued, the junta worked to unite the faculties, libraries, and instruments of the two schools. By redistributing course assignments, the junta had chairs for every professor. Classes, demonstrations, and the Thursday assemblies continued as usual. San Carlos had become a school of both medicine and surgery with remarkably little difficulty.

Unification was less successful in eliminating the traditional prejudices against the surgeon. The Academy of Medicine decided against offering membership to Gimbernat and his colleagues since "físicos" were not real physicians ("médicos").[44]

Enrollment soared as students flocked to San Carlos instead of the university. But their motives were questionable. During the 1799–1800 academic year the matriculation of Latin students doubled. At the same time the number of applications for licenses as physicians jumped as graduates discovered they were eligible. More than six times as many men became physicians in Madrid in 1800 as had done so only two years earlier.[45] Yet the sudden attraction of Latin surgery was probably due less to new respect for the subject than to the fact that the license received at graduation was more valuable. Did students flock to San Carlos rather than the universities because they sought a superior education or because they believed it was an easier route to becoming a physician? Certainly the dual license was desirable, but it seems equally certain that most students, faced with a choice between medicine and surgery, definitely preferred the former. When the experiment of unification came to an abrupt end in 1801 many San Carlos students transferred to universities to assure themselves a physician's license. Yet the prestige that accrued to San Carlos lived on, for, despite the dropouts, the total number of Latin students steadily climbed during the next few years. The prejudices of generations

42. AFM, Libro de Acuerdos para la Junta Superior, records forty-four such permissions between April 1 and June 30, 1800.

43. *Ibid.*, Orden de la Junta de la Facultad Reunida, Nov. 18, 1800.

44. Josef de Masdevall to Miguel Barnades, May 14, 1799, quoted in "Parte biográfica," in *Obras de Gimbernat*, I, 263–267.

45. AUC, Libro de Matrícula de Cirujanos Latinos (1787–1817); AGS, Dir. Gral. del Tesoro, Inventario 24, Leg. 977.

could not be eliminated by radical legal reforms, but they were substantially reduced.

The reformers also attempted to bring pharmacy, which had traditionally been regulated by the Protomedicato, into the united faculty. In November 1799 three pharmacists became members of the general board. Future pharmacists were now required to study at one of the royal colleges for two years in addition to the conventional two years of apprenticeship. However, a few months later the Crown created a separate board to regulate the profession.[46] Nevertheless, by 1800 everyone related to the healing arts in any way was to have had a common experience in one of the royal colleges. Its location in Madrid gave the College of San Carlos a preeminent position in medicine, surgery, and pharmacy alike.

Had medicine and surgery remained unified over several years the traditional contempt for the surgeon might have disappeared. This was not to be. In September 1801, barely two years after the creation of the united faculty, the conservative ministers that had replaced Urquijo and Cabellero put an end to the marriage of medicine and surgery and restored the healing arts to their previous dissected condition.[47]

The universities, quite naturally, had opposed unification from the start. Their outrage at being ignored and superseded was intensified by the reformers' total scorn and indifference for these traditional institutions. Gimbernat and his colleagues paid no attention to the progressive medical reformers at Salamanca. As a result, university protests ranged from scholarly criticisms of the San Carlos curriculum to paranoiac visions of dark conspiracies that would have Francophile doctors in Madrid plotting the subversion of all Spanish education.[48]

The sudden suppression of the united faculty, however, appears to have been as much the result of ministerial politics and personality conflicts as of the intense pressure from the traditional medical estab-

46. ARP, Leg. 691, *Concordia y Reales Ordenanzas para el Régimen y Gobierno de la Facultad de Farmacia, formadas con conocimiento de la Real Junta General de Gobierno de la Facultad Reunida* (Madrid, 1800), March 24, 1800.

47. *Real Cédula de S.M. y Señores del Consejo, por la cual se manda cesar la Junta General de Gobierno de la Facultad Reunida, se restablece el Protomedicato y que subsista la Junta Superior Gubernative de Farmacia con lo demás que se expresa* (Madrid, 1801), Sept. 28, 1801 (hereinafter cited as *Real Cédula por la cual se manda cesar la Facultad Reunida*). Copies exist in AHN, Consejos, Leg. 5444, Exp. 14, Parte 3, and Universidades, Sig. 1232.

Documents during these years make frequent reference to the additional colleges but do not describe their establishment.

48. Addy, *The Enlightenment in . . . Salamanca*, pp. 204–209.

lishment. In 1800 Pedro de Ceballos, who had close ties with influential conservatives and was more disposed to listen to their protests, came to power. Thus, the radical adventure rose and fell with the fortunes of Urquijo and Caballero.

The cédula that suppressed the united faculty referred to the "various difficulties" (*varios inconvenientes*) that had accompanied unification, but it did not elaborate upon their nature. It argued further that medicine and surgery were distinct sciences by nature, each of which had its own "well defined limits." Laws could not change this fact. It was superfluous to study both sciences. The school that taught both probably taught neither well. Such arguments were reminiscent of the opposition of the Protomedicato to autonomous schools of surgery when it had argued that an academic background was useless for a surgeon.

In the final analysis the advocates of unification probably attempted too much too fast. Their lack of thorough planning plus their underestimation of the opposition to the reform created as much frustration and confusion as progress. Moderate, tempered reform in eighteenth-century Spain was usually more productive in the long run. Yet it was unfortunate for the future of Spanish medicine and surgery that their unification became entwined with the bitter struggle between liberals and conservatives. For the next thirty years every liberal government that came to power would unite the two faculties, and every conservative government would separate them, almost as a matter of course. The question of unification became intimately linked to the French Revolution and Napoleon on the one hand and to traditional Spanish fueros on the other. Besides, after the restoration of the Protomedicato, Gimbernat lost his influence.

In any event, as a result of the royal cédula of September 28, 1801, three distinct jurisdictions, each of which was completely autonomous, replaced the united faculty. The restored Protomedicato again became responsible for licensing physicians and public health, although local courts of law retained jurisdiction over infractions of medical legislation. The academic training of physicians returned to the universities. At the same time the 1801 cédula established two separate superior administrative boards to govern surgery and pharmacy. Each board held jurisdiction over the royal colleges and licensing procedure in its respective field. Finally, the Crown again authorized new surgical colleges similar to San Carlos in Burgos, Santiago, and Salamanca.

The suppression of the united faculty did not, however, signify a departure from the established policies of restricting university autonomy and reducing the inferior position of surgery. In 1804, in an effort to underline the "separate but equal" status of the three branches, the Crown replaced the Protomedicato with a Superior Administrative Board of Medicine. Like its two counterparts, the new board was responsible for all medical education, including the right to intervene in the medical faculties of the universities.[49] Thus, the return to the previous organization was still a victory of sorts for Gimbernat, since surgery as a separate but equal division of the profession was preferable to its subordination to medicine.

The 1801 cédula also restored San Carlos and the School of Practical Medicine to their former status as distinct institutions. The juntas of the two schools carefully returned student files, library books, and anatomical instruments to their respective institutions. Classes continued as usual. The Superior Board of Surgery reassumed its former role. San Carlos continued to certify surgeons for want of any instructions to the contrary. Meanwhile, Antonio Gimbernat succeeded Pedro Custodio Gutiérrez as First Surgeon of His Majesty. The faculties of both schools easily adjusted to their prior status.

But San Carlos students were less amenable to the new condition. Young men who had looked forward to practicing medicine suddenly found themselves destined to become mere surgeons. Many were understandably upset. During the next few years many San Carlos students decided to transfer to a university. The faculty of San Carlos, moreover, was irritated to discover that so many students had no interest in surgery but had simply "used" San Carlos to become physicians. Accordingly, it refused to certify that any student who had not completed the course had studied at San Carlos. The student thus had to repeat several years of study. The San Carlos faculty argued with some justification that the curriculum of the school was a complete course; individual classes had little value except as part of the complete program. Moreover, the San Carlos curriculum was "based on other principles, and more solid fundamentals," than that of a university.[50] To certify a student who had not taken the full course would

49. ARP, Leg. 691. *Real Cédula de S.M. y Señores del Consejo por la qual se manda formar una Junta Superior de Medicina que vele sobre esta enseñanza, sus progresos y profesores, baxo las reglas que se expresan* (Madrid, 1804), Feb. 5, 1804 (hereinafter cited as *Real Cédula sobre la Junta de Medicina*).

50. AHN, Consejos, Leg. 5445, Expediente de Juan Rodríguez del Piño, Informe del

defeat the very principles for which San Carlos stood. Many of the students appealed to the Council of Castile. The Council, angered at the arrogance of the San Carlos faculty, readily ordered the certifications every time, despite the protests of the college.

Meanwhile, the San Carlos faculty, convinced that its college was better than a university and embittered at being returned to an inferior status, tried to continue to turn out graduates who were both physicians and surgeons. The 1799 reform had altered the six-year surgical course so that the sixth year was devoted to the clinic in internal medicine. After the restoration, the faculty simply offered a five-year course and then allowed its students to attend the School of Practical Medicine. Thus, after seven years a student could receive both licenses as under the united faculty without ever entering a university. In a further display of arrogance, San Carlos gave its graduates a license of medical surgeon (*cirujano-médico*).

The faculty apparently hoped that such duplicity would lead to skilled surgeons who were licensed to practice medicine. However, by the beginning of the 1803–1804 academic year it began to realize that students were taking advantage of the device to become physicians. This thwarted the college's basic purpose of training skilled surgeons since, for the most part, only the romance students actually intended to practice surgery. Gimbernat, now president of the Superior Board, was particularly disturbed.

For the next few weeks rumors circulated that San Carlos students might be unable to become physicians and that the course might be restored to six years as provided in the 1795 statutes. Many of the students, fearful for their career plans, were angry and upset. On November 19, having decided to take action, the students began the college's first strike. For the next five days no matriculated students attended class, although a few auditors continued coming. At the weekly exercises the following Thursday, after José Ribes finished reading a lecture on a kidney disease, the students confronted the assembled faculty. They declared that they had come to San Carlos to become medical surgeons and demanded that they be allowed to do so. Sev-

---

Colegio de San Carlos, Oct. 10, 1801. This legajo contains several similar requests from San Carlos students. AUC, Libro de Matrícula de Cirujanos Latinos (1787–1817), lists many students who left.

The policy of withholding credit from those who did not complete the course began in June 1801, probably in response to rumors that the united faculty might be suppressed. (AFM, Libro de Acuerdos [1787–1804], Junta of June 25, 1801).

eral students reiterated the arguments for a united faculty and added that as mere surgeons they would not be able to support their families adequately. The faculty listened patiently but claimed this was a question for the Superior Board to decide. The students then decided to petition the Crown directly. During the next few days they slowly returned to classes.[51]

The students did not have to wait long for an answer. Between the Crown's determination to suppress any remnants of the united faculty and Gimbernat's fear for the future of Latin surgery, the students had little chance. On December 1, 1803, after consulting Gimbernat, the Crown declared that henceforth only graduates of university medical faculties could become physicians, and only graduates of surgical colleges could become surgeons.[52] Five months later (May 1804), new statutes for all surgical colleges confirmed the demise of medicine at San Carlos. Despite the efforts of the San Carlos faculty and student body, the separation of surgery and medicine was now complete.

Although Gimbernat and the San Carlos faculty were disappointed that surgery was once again separate from medicine, the suppression of the united faculty did not signify the end of reform. The age of Spanish reform ended with the reign of Ferdinand VII in 1814, not with the death of Charles III in 1788. Substantial changes that threatened established interests became unlikely, but moderate revision continued. Indeed, the intense planning during the years preceding the French invasion was reminiscent of the intense activity during the reign of Charles III. Godoy himself took an active interest in public health, giving his support to measures designed to improve urban sanitation and disease control.[53] The three boards that regulated the medical profession were composed of progressive individuals. One of the first actions of the Board of Medicine was to promote universal vaccination. The Crown in 1804 required every hospital to vaccinate anyone who requested it without charge.[54] However, the board focused most of its attention on improving the universities and restoring some order to the chaos created by the united faculty. The 1801 cédula had restored the monopoly of the universities on the education of physicians. At the same time the Crown had ordered all faculties of medicine to include

51. AFM, Libro de Acuerdos (1787–1804), Juntas of Oct. 13, Nov. 24, 1804.

52. *Ibid.*, Junta of Dec. 1, 1803.

53. In his *Memorias*, II, 64, Godoy declares that public health was his "major concern" in 1805.

54. *Nov. Rec.*, VII, xxxviii, 9.

anatomy, experimental physics, and clinical training in their curriculum and to begin revising their entire plan of studies.[55] In 1804, in keeping with its policy of complete separation, the Crown suppressed all surgical training in the universities. As before, however, university graduates had to study two years at the Madrid School of Practical Medicine.[56]

The universities varied in their response to the call for further reform. The medical faculty at Salamanca acted immediately after receiving the 1801 cédula. Using its 1789 proposals as a basis, it quickly drew up a new curriculum and forwarded it to Madrid.[57] The Crown approved it in 1804. The new curriculum provided for a six-year course of study in which the student logically progressed from anatomy and physiology to pathology, materia médica, and internal diseases. Every student frequently performed anatomical exercises on a cadaver. The last two years consisted primarily of clinical training, thereby alleviating the need for Salamancan students to attend the clinic in Madrid. The reform required all students to have studied experimental physics before matriculating and to study chemistry during their first year. The natural sciences were becoming increasingly important for future physicians. All in all, the new curriculum was virtually identical to that of San Carlos. Even the rationale and syllabus for the individual courses were the same. Thus, in 1804, the significant reforms advocated by Gimbernat were finally realized in medical education despite the defeat of its unification with surgery. The universities were far more capable of progressive innovation than he had believed.

Not every university was so eager to change. At Alcalá conditions were "in a state of decadence and confusion," which the rector blamed on the reforms of Charles III.[58] The university had never completely accepted the reforms of the 1770s and had done nothing to implement clinical practice or establish a single course in botany as required by the 1801 restoration. When in 1805 a young substitute professor complained of this to the Crown, the cloister merely apologized for his

55. *Real Cédula por la cual se manda cesar la Facultad Reunida.*

56. ARP, Leg. 691, *Real Cédula sobre la Junta de Medicina*; AFM, Libro de Acuerdos (1787–1804), Junta of April 29, 1804. Salamanca was permitted to offer its own clinical training.

57. AHN, Consejos, Leg. 5468, Parte 1, Exp. 58, Plan de Estudios de la Facultad de Medicina de la Universidad de Salamanca, 1804. For the background to its acceptance, see Addy, *The Enlightenment in . . . Salamanca*, pp. 211–214.

58. AHN, Consejos, Leg. 5438, Exp. 3, Representación de Mariano Martín Esperanza, Rector, Feb. 13, 1805.

unseemly requests.[59] The faculty as a whole seemed bereft of any initiative. The medical faculty waited for word from the Superior Board before doing a thing. The rector of the university requested that the Council of Castile stage an official inspection (*visita*) in order to learn first-hand the evils produced by reforms his university had yet to implement. The fiscal of the Council, while not agreeing on the causes of the university's problems, readily agreed that an inspection would be a good idea.[60] This "visit" began two years later but was never completed, for a more general reform of all universities was impending.

While the universities contended with their new situation, the royal commission, first established in 1800 to standardize all medical education, set to work drawing up a standard curriculum for all the colleges of surgery. Although Gimbernat remained a member, his influence declined after 1801 and the commission ignored many of his suggestions. The commission's deliberations resulted in the ordinances of 1804, which placed all colleges of surgery under the Superior Board of Surgery and established a standard curriculum. The new entrance requirements that permitted Scholastic philosophy and the omission of courses in the natural sciences marked a step backward for San Carlos. For the first time the royal college was less progressive than the University of Salamanca.

The new statutes also confirmed that aspect of the united faculty whereby the colleges themselves accredited practitioners. Henceforth, each college was responsible not only for the academic progress of its own students but for conducting examinations and granting licenses for all practitioners except physicians and pharmacists. In essence, the schools assumed the traditional function of the Protomedicato. The same statutes radically revised the examinations themselves.

The licensing examinations were time-consuming affairs for faculty and student alike.[61] Latin students automatically received the degree of bachelor of surgery upon successfully completing their fifth year. After the sixth year, however, they had to pass a thorough examination

59. AHN, Consejos, Leg. 5438, Exp. 4, Memorial de Manuel Arroyo, Feb. 18, 1805; Informe del Claustro Pleno, May 29, 1805.

60. AHN, Consejos, Leg. 5438, Exp. 4, Informe del Claustro Pleno, May 29, 1805; Exp. 3, Representación de Mariano Martín Esperanza, Rector, Feb. 13, 1805; Dictamen del Fiscal, April 4, 1805.

61. The examinations are minutely described in *Ordenanzas Generales* (1804), Cap. XVI. *Nov. Rec.*, VIII, xii, 12, is an excerpt.

before receiving their licentiate. The examination was divided into two parts, theory and practice. For the first, the student had to answer questions, some of which could relate to internal medicine, posed by three faculty members. For the second part the student had to perform successfully an assigned operation on a cadaver in order to prove his "manual dexterity." Finally, he was brought to an unfamiliar patient suffering from a "mixed disease." After half an hour he had to describe the patient's malady and what he would do to cure him. The two-part practical exercise was a radical departure from the traditional emphasis on memorization alone.

The examinations for the other positions were similar, if less thorough. The potential romance surgeon had an oral exam and the same practical exam, except that the questions involved only "external diseases." Both the requirements and the examinations made a sharp distinction between Latin and romance surgeons. The new format also continued the title of "bleeder" (*sangrador*). To be licensed, an applicant needed three years of practice plus an examination at one of the surgical colleges. The theoretical part consisted of questions on the blood vessels, conditions that called for bleeding, and the pulling of teeth. For the practical exercise, he had to perform a phlebotomy. The applicant for the license of midwife, besides passing the exam, also had to have assisted a licensed midwife for three years after having taken the San Carlos course. Only married women could apply. The Superior Board was to publish a handbook for women in rural areas to study in preparation for the exam.[62] In every case the three examiners voted by depositing a white (passed) or black (failed) ball in an urn. To pass, one needed two favorable votes. The student could retake his exam twice.

Candidates for all licenses also had to document their limpieza de sangre. Apparently the documents were easily forged and the surgical colleges increasingly careless in examining them. On several occasions the Crown demanded that the schools act more cautiously in certifying the documents. In 1807 San Carlos was ordered to check with local officials in the village from which the applicant came if there was the slightest doubt of the veracity of his statements.[63]

Although the colleges charged no tuition, the fees for the examination were not inconsequential. The fee for surgeons was 2,500 reales, or more than the stipend of a resident student for sixteen months.

62. I have seen no record of whether or not the handbook was ever published.
63. AUC, Libro de Ordenes, Oficio of Nov. 23, 1807.

Bleeders had to pay 2,000 reales and a midwife 800. Each examiner received twenty reales of the fee, while the rest went to support the colleges of surgery.

The new statutes also were designed to cope with the demoralizing jealousy and bitterness of the Latin surgeon toward the physician, and of the romance surgeon toward the Latin surgeon. The former was a particularly thorny issue since most of the San Carlos faculty and student body felt that the distinction was unjustified. As more capable young men returned to universities, the caliber of the San Carlos student body declined. Even the prestige of the school itself suffered. By 1805, despite the new statutes, so many students failed to meet the strict standards of the examiners that the secretary of grace and justice inquired as to the reason of the "decadence" of surgery in general and San Carlos in particular. Without a moment's hesitation, the faculty attributed the "decadence" to the suppression of the united faculty. One could not criticize young men for seeking the career with "more honors."[64]

The authors of the new statutes and, later, the Board of Surgery were concerned but not willing to reunite the two professions. Instead they tried a compromise. If "honor" was at the root of the problem, additional honors for surgeons could help solve it. Accordingly, they reestablished the academic degree of doctor of surgery.

The degree of doctor of surgery originated with the statutes of 1795 in order to give surgery "its due honor and approbation . . . and to raise it from the unjust depression and disdain" that retarded its progress. It enabled surgeons to win "the honors, distinctions, and prerogatives of those who receive the highest degree in the universities."[65] An elaborate ceremony accompanied the conferring of this degree. First, the candidate himself delivered an oration in Latin. Then his sponsor spoke eloquently of his merits and accomplishments. Colorful processions began and concluded the ceremony. Despite the pomp, any Latin surgeon willing to pay the fee of 1,500 reales could become doctor of surgery.

The establishment of the degree was of benefit in a society so conscious of titles and privileges. The 1804 statutes made a further concession to surgery in order to make it more attractive to status-conscious young men. Henceforth, any doctor of surgery could obtain a license

64. The Secretary's *oficio* is quoted in AUC, Libro de Acuerdos (1804–1810), Junta of Oct. 10, 1805. The Juntas of Oct. 14, Oct. 17, 1805, contain the school's response.

65. *Ordenanzas* (1795), Parte Tercera, Cap. XIV.

to practice internal medicine as a physician, or médico, by studying at the Royal School of Practical Medicine for two years and passing the licensing examination. Thus, the doctorate effectively enabled San Carlos students to circumvent the laws that made university study a prerequisite to practicing medicine. In 1805 the Crown allowed San Carlos graduates who entered the army to practice medicine without the two years of clinical training. By 1807 a student could receive the doctorate at the same time he received his license.[66]

The authors of the ordinances of 1804 also tried to bridge the gap between Latin and romance surgeons. Now that romance students also had to attend a surgical college, both classes had similar educational backgrounds. The romance student spent five years taking the same courses as his Latin colleagues. However, the romance student could receive his license at the end of those five years, whereas the Latin student had to study an additional year of "mixed diseases." Thus, the latter was superior only in his medical background. Nevertheless, only a Latin surgeon could hope to win a position of prestige in a hospital, the military, or in the colleges themselves.

Clearly the romance surgeon differed from his Latin colleague only in his lack of a bachelor of arts degree (the Latin, logic, and sciences required for matriculation) and that sixth year on internal diseases. In August 1804 the Crown declared that any romance surgeon could become a Latin surgeon by simply completing the requirements he lacked and taking the exam. He could study the arts courses anywhere.[67] However, the faculty of San Carlos, always concerned for the order in which subjects were taken, apparently hesitated to grant the Latin licenses. The Superior Board frequently had to support specific applicants by reminding the school of its obligation.[68]

Despite these efforts to make Latin surgery more easily attainable, romance surgeons continued to outnumber Latin surgeons in both the San Carlos student body and in the licenses granted by the college. For example, between 1810 and 1816 some sixty to one hundred romance students attended San Carlos each year, while Latin students never numbered more than fifteen. On the other hand, far fewer romance students completed the course and received licenses. In 1816 the school licensed eight Latin surgeons but only twenty-three ro-

66. AFM, Libro de Representaciones, Ordenes, etc., Reales ordenes, Nov. 15, 1805, Aug. 14, 1807.

67. *Ibid.*, Real orden, Aug. 14, 1804.

68. For example, AUC, Libro de Acuerdos (1804–1810), Juntas of Aug. 23, 1804; Dec. 5, 1805; AUC, Libro de Ordenes, Oficio of Aug. 20, 1805.

mance surgeons.[69] Knowledge of the Latin language was probably a stumbling block for some. On the other hand, the student with a Latin background was probably better prepared to embark successfully on five or six very demanding years.

The frequent modifications, difficult enough for experts to follow, must have meant total confusion for the general public. Some romance surgeons took advantage of the situation by flaunting their San Carlos documents and claiming to be Latin surgeons deserving of higher fees. Such frauds occurred so frequently that the Superior Board finally ordered that only those who promised to return to their native village to practice could be licensed in romance surgery.[70] Though difficult to enforce, the order relegated the less-educated surgeon to rural villages, while better-trained practitioners would hopefully come to monopolize the profession in population centers.

Nevertheless, by 1807 the surgeons of San Carlos had succeeded in making its approach to the training of medical practitioners the norm throughout Spain. Although the formal distinctions between physician and surgeon persisted, differences in their education had all but disappeared. The progressives not only set the standards for education but completely controlled the licensing requirements as well. Only institutional jealousies and popular prejudices continued to prevent surgery from receiving the respect and dignity it now so richly deserved.

In 1807 the government of Godoy decided to undertake still another full-scale reform of professional and higher education. The brunt of this new effort fell on the universities, which received a new standardized curriculum in July of 1807.[71] Despite the efforts of the more liberal universities such as Salamanca, the 1807 statutes were solely the product of government personnel.[72] They began by suppressing eleven universities that were either so decadent that reform seemed impossible or too short of funds to continue in operation. Among the remaining eleven universities, those that lacked the necessary funds or facilities to teach medicine were to abolish that faculty.

69. AUC, Libro de Matrícula de Cirujanos Latinos (1787–1817); Libro de Matrículas de Romancistas (1800—); Libro Tercero de Reválides (1816–1820). The AUC does not have the complete collection of this type of material. Accurate statistics are difficult since identifications of the candidates vary from year to year.

70. AUC, Libro de Ordenes, Oficio of Aug. 18, 1806.

71. AHN, Universidades, Sig. 1232, *Real Cédula de S.M. y Señores del Consejo, por la qual se reduce el número de las Universidades literarias del Reyno; se agregan las suprimidas a las que quedan, según su localidad; y se manda observar en ellas el Plan de Estudios aprobado para la de Salamanca en la forma que se expresa* (Madrid, 1807), July 12, 1807.

72. Addy, *The Enlightenment in . . . Salamanca*, pp. 231–232.

Most of the new statutes were devoted to elaborating a new curriculum for all Spanish universities. Theology, arts, and law underwent substantial change. Mathematics and experimental physics became a standard part of the arts course.

As university reform neared completion, the Crown created another commission to review "the structure and education of the faculty of the art of curing." The eight-member board included Gimbernat and two San Carlos professors.[73] The new commission was the culmination of the trend whereby medical and surgical education were together considered as one aspect of the medical profession rather than as part of the university. That a commission existed apart from the separate administrative boards suggested that a united faculty was once again a real possibility.

The invasion by Napoleon interrupted the work of the commission, and the debate over a united faculty became lost in the difficult years that followed. Yet it is to the credit of Godoy that his government continued its efforts to modernize Spanish education until the very end. Indeed, history has been unfair to the government of Manuel Godoy. It has praised the reforms under Charles III but has pictured the reign of Charles IV as a time of political intrigue and ideological hassles. Such a picture is correct but not complete. To be sure, theology, philosophy, and law were potentially explosive, and perhaps reformers in these fields had to behave more carefully. In nonpolitical disciplines such as medicine, however, the history of the College of San Carlos clearly proves that during the reign of Charles IV reform, experiment, and progress continued unabated. Within San Carlos the period between 1788 and 1808 marked the culmination of a century of advances in medicine and surgery. As the French armies crossed the Pyrenees, Spain could be justifiably proud of its medical education.

73. AFM, Libro de Representaciones, Ordenes, etc., Real orden, July 23, 1807; Agustín de Gimbernat, *Noticia de Gimbernat, pp.* 55–57; Salcedo de Ginestal, "Parte biográfica," in *Obras de Gimbernat*, I, 290–291.

CHAPTER VII

# SAN CARLOS, MEDICAL EDUCATION, AND POLITICAL TURMOIL, 1808–1833

THE TORTUROUS ROAD to further reform in the education of physicians and surgeons came to an abrupt stop with the invasion by Napoleon Bonaparte. By March 1808 more than 100,000 French soldiers were marching toward Madrid. Agents of the future Ferdinand VII, who was eager to seize his father's crown, used the French invasion to fan the fires of popular hatred toward Manuel Godoy, the "Prince of Peace." To the religious Spaniard, only Godoy was more despicable than the atheistic French. The hated minister who had made a cuckold of his king was now a traitor to his nation.

The king always spent March at Aranjuez, accompanied by his ministers and household. During this particular March a lively debate took place on whether or not the king should flee south in the face of the advancing French. Meanwhile, a large crowd of soldiers and hangers-on, some curious, some angry, gathered outside the palace. Ferdinand's agents helped keep tensions high. On the evening of March 17 the mood of the crowd turned ugly. Around midnight the mob attacked Godoy's house in search of the hated Prince of Peace. Godoy barely escaped with his life, hiding himself under some old rugs, where he remained for the next thirty-six hours. The next morning the king dismissed his minister in the vain hope of satisfying the mob. Faced with still worse rioting two nights later, King Charles IV decided to abdicate in favor of his son, Ferdinand. The crowd was ecstatic, but the joy was short-lived. Two days later General Murat led his French troops into Madrid. It was not only the end of a reign; it was the end of the eighteenth century in Spain.

For the next twenty years Spain was the prisoner of invasions, civil wars, revolutions, and repression. At the College of San Carlos political matters forced questions of pedagogy into the background. The fine points of curriculum reform and examination procedure seemed insignificant in comparison with the weightier questions that would determine the very future of Spain. It is to the credit of the college's staff that the work of education continued at all. Indeed, San Carlos emerged from the turmoil virtually unscathed.

The San Carlos faculty received formal notification of the dismissal of Godoy and the abdication of Charles IV on March 31, 1808. As usual, the secretary simply recorded the communication without noting the reaction of the professors. Meanwhile, French troops were already in Madrid and in need of medical facilities. On April 2 the school received a royal order to make the anatomical theater into a hospital ward. The professors were to allow their students to miss classes so they might care for additional patients. The order specified that the school was to do everything possible to insure the French received proper medical care.[1] Nevertheless, all classes and the weekly lectures continued for the rest of the month.

On April 10 Ferdinand VII left Madrid for his ill-fated interview with Napoleon at Bayonne. In Madrid hatred toward the French increased with the frustrations and humiliation of a foreign occupation. Finally the pent-up emotions of the Madrid populace exploded in anti-French rioting on May 2. French troops fired into the crowd. Spanish partisans killed French soldiers. Yet a poorly armed civilian population was no match for Napoleon's regulars, and order was quickly restored through summary executions and overwhelming force. General Murat installed himself in the Royal Palace. As the repression continued, the San Carlos junta met on May 6 and decided to suspend all classes for the time being.

Unlike the populace of Madrid, the Spanish bureaucracy accepted French rule with little protest. While Napoleon completed his plans for his latest acquisition, many public officials in Madrid paid their respects to their new ruler, General Murat. The Council of Castile, maintaining its traditional posture of supporting established authority, all but ignored Ferdinand's pleas to resist. Instead, the Council routinely published Murat's decrees.

In early June, Napoleon declared his brother Joseph king of Spain. The new monarch immediately appointed his cabinet. Luis Mariano de Urquijo, the liberal former First Secretary from 1798 to 1800, became minister of state. Pedro Ceballos, who had replaced Urquijo in 1800

1. AUC, Libro de Acuerdos (1804–1810), Juntas of March 31, April 2, 1808. The French arrived in Madrid on March 23. Ferdinand VII arrived a day later.

and had also served Ferdinand during his brief rule, became minister of foreign affairs. The other two members, Francisco Cabarrús and Gonzalo O'Farril, also served Ferdinand as minister of finance and minister of war, respectively. O'Farril was also a member of the Council of Castile. Joseph himself entered Madrid on July 20. The people of Madrid gave him an unenthusiastic reception. Yet, except for the monarch himself, the faces of the governors of Spain had not changed much.[2]

The San Carlos faculty conducted no further business until May 24, when it met to consider a request from General Murat to reopen the school. Since the Superior Administrative Board endorsed the request, the school readily complied.[3] The year ended without incident. Only one professor, Pedro Castelló, resigned in protest to the French occupation and retreated to Mallorca. The Superior Board also continued to function as usual. Its membership, including Antonio Gimbernat, remained the same. Thus, except for an unanticipated vacation in May, surgical education was unaffected by the dramatic events that occurred during the spring of 1808. Members of the Superior Board and the faculty chose to accept what seemed inevitable rather than risk losing the fruits of decades of work.

Although life in Madrid had returned to normal by early summer, word of the May uprising had spread rapidly throughout the peninsula. Spanish patriots almost everywhere rallied to throw out the intruders. In mid-July they defeated a large French army at Bailén. On August 1 Joseph and his French troops withdrew from Madrid, leaving the city and San Carlos under the rule of, first, the indecisive Council of Castile, and, after September 25, the new patriotic Junta Central, whose president was the aging reformer, the Conde de Floridablanca.

The San Carlos junta did not meet until August 28, when the professors agreed to serve in various ad hoc infirmaries throughout the city should the fighting return. There was no mention of the school's previous cooperation with the French. Two weeks later the junta decided to dispense with the annual examinations. It was also unsure whether to hold the annual religious celebration in honor of Saints Cosmas and Damian on September 28. The Superior Board, anxious to return to normal, advised the school to hold the observance but, as funds were short, to contribute less than usual to the preacher.[4]

2. Lovett, *Napoleon*, I, 120–132; Miguel Artola, *Los orígenes de la España contemporánea* (2 vols.; Madrid, 1949), I, 109–114.

3. AUC, Libro de Acuerdos (1804–1810), Junta of May 24, 1808.

4. AUC, Libro de Ordenes, Oficio of Sept. 6, 1808; Libro de Acuerdos (1804–1810), Juntas of Aug. 28, Sept. 15, 1808.

The future appeared promising during October and November. Floridablanca named a cabinet that included the ubiquitous Pedro Ceballos, who had now decided to place his fortunes with the patriotic resistance. San Carlos opened as usual on October 1 with a formal lecture. Classes commenced the following morning. The junta and Superior Board returned to their consideration of specific student problems. On October 20 all patients were removed from the anatomical theater.[5]

Napoleon had not so easily forgotten Spain. In early November he himself led an army of more than 250,000 men into Spain to subdue that defiant nation. Madrid capitulated on December 3, after a brave but futile defense. Napoleon quickly initiated his policy of liberalism by the sword. In rapid succession he abolished feudal rights, suppressed the Inquisition, and reduced the number of religious houses. In a few days he accomplished what generations of Spanish reformers had not dared to do. Few Spaniards, however, applauded the foreign conqueror.

Since the French occupied the capital city until 1813, Madrid could not and did not participate in the struggle for independence and the efforts to establish a liberal constitutional regime. Madrileños had little choice but to make the best of a difficult situation, for French troops were present in force.

Joseph Napoleon returned to Madrid in February 1809, intent on making his reign permanent. He was determined to fill the bureaucracy with men he could trust and to dismiss the uncommitted who simply wished to hold on to their jobs.[6] He was equally determined to initiate substantial reform in the kingdom his brother had given him. Thus, he gathered a small number of dedicated Frenchified liberals, the *afrancesados*, who saw in Joseph the means of obtaining those reforms for which they had worked so hard for so many decades. As minister of state the new monarch chose Mariano Luis de Urquijo, who used his position to implement the reforms that he had seen frustrated a decade earlier.

Soon after Joseph returned to Madrid the surgeons of San Carlos had to decide whether to cooperate again with the French. In late February Joseph issued a decree ordering all government employees to take an oath of allegiance to his new government. The Superior Board

5. AUC, Libro de Acuerdos (1804–1810), Juntas of Oct. 1, Oct. 13, Oct. 20, Oct. 27, 1808.

6. Letter from the Comte de la Forest, Madrid, Aug. 20, 1809, No. 144, in *Correspondance du Comte de la Forest*, ed. Geoffroy de Grandmaison (7 vols.; Paris, 1908), II, 377.

routinely forwarded the decree to San Carlos. The San Carlos faculty agreed to take the oath on February 24, only a week after the decree was issued. The precise text of the oath, which called for complete dedication to "the well-being of the Nation and the glory of the king in conformity with the Constitution," arrived in May.[7] The faculty secretary, perhaps fearful of future repercussions, did not record whether the professors actually took the oath. It may be presumed that they did.

Apparently other government officials hesitated to do the same. In August Joseph discharged all government employees and required them to apply for their positions anew. The Superior Board of Surgery, however, enjoyed exemption from this requirement. As a result of petitions from the board, Joseph declared all San Carlos professors similarly exempt a month later. The entire faculty agreed to continue its duties under the intruder government.[8]

The minutes of the junta say nothing, as is natural, of the inevitable arguments and doubts that must have occurred in response to these royal decrees. While so much of Spain was up in arms, the members of the Superior Board and the San Carlos faculty pledged allegiance to the alien regime and did everything possible to carry on as usual. There are several possible explanations for the surgeons' cooperation with the French. Some may simply have accepted the interlopers and decided to cooperate in order to hold on to their positions. Overt opposition could have resulted in unemployment. However, the dedication and concern most of the affected surgeons had exhibited in the past make it unlikely that personal motives alone were responsible.

Most of the surgeons, including Antonio Gimbernat, probably offered no opposition in order not to destroy surgical education during the occupation. They saw themselves as scientists, not politicians. This instance was not the first in which they had cooperated with despicable individuals and it would not be the last. Politics was not their affair. Gimbernat, for example, was willing to pay any price in order to continue to promote surgical training. As long as the French showed themselves interested in educational reforms, he saw no reason to oppose them. Overt opposition would only bring about the closing of San Carlos. As early as December 17, 1808, only two weeks after Madrid had fallen a second time to the French, the Superior Board decided not

7. AUC, Libro de Acuerdos (1804–1810), Juntas of Feb. 24, May 19, 1808. The constitution referred to was drawn up in Bayonne under Napoleon's supervision. Under it Joseph became, in theory, Spain's first constitutional monarch.

8. *Ibid.*, Juntas of Aug. 24, Aug. 28, Sept. 18, 1809.

to resist the occupation and risk complete suppression. Faced with the threat that the French might order the school to evacuate the Hospital General in order to make more room available for wounded soldiers, the board ordered the school to open immediately in order to convince the French of the school's value and to persuade them to give it financial support.[9]

In addition to such pragmatic considerations, it is quite possible that some surgeons were afrancesados, willing collaborators with the French. Many had studied in France. Others admired the medical and educational reforms of the French Revolution. Indeed, the Napoleonic style was not unlike the "enlightened despotism" of Charles III that had served them so well—reform through centralized authority. The afrancesados were committed to such reform without violence. In the words of one historian, "The *ilustrado* of the reign of Charles III was the *afrancesado* of 1808."[10] Joseph presented himself as a reformer committed to making education more applicable to the real needs of society, and he showed little sympathy for traditional privilege. Thus, Gimbernat and his colleagues may have seen the French as a new ally in their efforts to modernize Spanish education. Perhaps their dedication to science outweighed their love of country. Or perhaps theirs was a greater patriotism that demanded their continued service to the people of Spain regardless of politics. War only worsened the terrible shortage of trained surgeons.

The French invasion also posed more immediate problems. In December 1808 the junta pointed out to the Superior Board that they had not received their salaries for several months. Four months later the professors pleaded with the board to remedy the situation so that they would be able to subsist. Finally the board gave its permission for the professors to take a portion of the amount owed them from the funds held in the school. This apparently enabled the professors to survive until examination fees refilled the school's coffers. However, due to the chaotic financial situation, the school was still dangerously short of funds. The junta was unable to answer the desperate pleas of the school's porters for enough money on which to live. In 1812 there were insufficient funds to hold an oposición to fill a vacant chair of anatomy.

9. *Ibid.*, Junta of Dec. 17, 1808. For Gimbernat's motives, see Salcedo y Ginestal, "Parte biográfica," in *Obras de Gimbernat*, I, 291–300. By this time Gimbernat was partially blind and frequently bedridden.

10. Miguel Artola, *Los Afrancesados* (Madrid, 1958), p. 41. For Napoleon's educational reforms in France, see L. P. Williams, "Science, Education, and Napoleon," *Isis*, XLVII (1956), 369–382.

Perhaps the dire financial straits of the school were best illustrated when the Superior Board gave the school permission to melt down two gold medals for operating expenses.[11]

Despite the financial crises, San Carlos continued to hold classes, examinations, and the weekly meetings of the junta. The collection of anatomical pieces continued to grow. Occasional disciplinary problems in the clinic seemed to further underline the return to normality. The intruder government even continued the practice of submitting manuscripts relating to medicine to the San Carlos faculty before publication. Only the weekly public exercises were affected by the occupation. After much discussion the junta decided to discontinue them during the occupation in order to avoid incidents. Since they frequently lasted into the evening, persons leaving the exercises would risk robbery and arrest for breaking the curfew.[12]

The government of Joseph Napoleon not only encouraged schools and institutes to continue to function but also endeavored to provide Spain with the educational benefits of the French Revolution. Indeed, Joseph's policy of uniformity and commitment to "useful knowledge" was not unlike that of Charles III and Charles IV. Many of his reforms also resembled those of the liberal Cortes and finally became permanent during the reign of Isabel II.[13]

During the autumn of 1809 Joseph created a Board of Public Instruction (*Junta de Instrucción Pública*) to supervise all education in occupied Spain. Never before had Spain witnessed such a body. The new board immediately demanded a report from every school on its structure, objectives, and shortcomings. The decree sent to San Carlos requested information on the state of medicine as a whole. Why, asked the board, was Spanish surgical education falling far short of the high standards set by the school's founders? The board requested the junta to be completely candid in its response. San Carlos also had to submit monthly reports on its academic and financial status. The Superior Board of Surgery also fell under the jurisdiction of the powerful new commission.[14]

11. AUC, Libro de Acuerdos (1804–1810), Juntas of Dec. 17, 1808; April 16, April 27, 1809; March 2, Dec. 10, 1810; Feb. 7, 1812.

12. *Ibid.*, Juntas of April 27, Sept. 22, 1809; April 5, Nov. 19, 1810; AUC, Libro de Ordenes, Oficio of Nov. 12, 1810.

13. On education in occupied Madrid, see Eugenio Sarrablo Aguareles, *La vida en Madrid durante la ocupación francesa de 1808 a 1813* (Zaragoza, 1964), pp. 228–230. The Madrid city government subsidized many schools.

14. AUC, Libro de Acuerdos (1804–1810), Juntas of Dec. 8, Dec. 22, 1809; Nov. 29, 1810; AFM, Libro de Representaciones, Ordenes, etc., Ordenes del Ministerio de la Interior, Oct. 23, Dec. 15, 1809.

San Carlos apparently met the rigid standards of the new government. The minister of war, Gonzalo O'Farril, attended the annual inaugural ceremonies in 1810. After a thorough tour of the library, the exhibits, and the clinic, he listened to the opening lecture, aptly entitled "The Physician in Wartime." The school secretary noted that O'Farril was very impressed. The efforts San Carlos made to please the new government were not in vain. Three days later the junta received a message from the minister of the interior noting his pleasure with "the zeal and ability" of the professors. More important, the communication promised regular financial assistance for the college.[15]

Not every institution of learning was acceptable to the French. The University of Salamanca was such an example. The local French commander, General Paul Thiebault, was so interested in educational reform that he imposed his own plan of studies upon the university. Although he left medicine as it was, the French commander expanded the natural sciences, introduced the Napoleonic code to legal studies, curtailed theology, and suppressed the faculty of canons entirely. He also placed the university under civil law.[16]

In early 1811 the Napoleonic government reunited the separate jurisdictions of medicine, surgery, and pharmacy into one Supreme Council of Health (*Consejo Supremo de Sanidad*) under the Ministry of the Interior. Spanish medical leaders had apparently allied themselves with Urquijo to win unification; the royal decree declared the action was in response to petitions from the three boards. Using identical arguments to those of Gimbernat and his colleagues a decade earlier, the decree argued that all medicine was the same in "principles" and "objectives." Antonio Gimbernat became president of the new council.[17] From his point of view, the reign of Joseph Napoleon served surgery well.

The fall of Madrid, however, had not led to the fall of Spain. While Joseph ruled in the capital, loyal Spaniards continued their struggle for independence with British aid in the south. In unoccupied Spain a succession of councils and juntas governed in the name of Ferdinand VII. Liberals took advantage of the absence of any central authority to plan

15. AUC, Libro de Acuerdos (1804–1810), Juntas of Oct. 1, Oct. 4, 1810.

16. AHN, Consejos, Leg. 5468, Parte 1, Exp. 58, Informe General sobre la Universidad de Salamanca por el General de Divisiòn Thiebault, 1811.

17. AUC, Libro de Acuerdos (1810–1816), Juntas of Feb. 19, Feb. 26, 1811; AFM, Libro de Representaciones, Ordenes, etc., Reales Ordenes, Jan. 28, 1811, Feb. 1, 1812. Significantly, Mariano Luis de Urquijo, who had sponsored unification in 1799, served Joseph Napoleon as minister of state.

widespread reform, all the while deluding themselves into believing that popular hatred of the French signified support for a more liberal state. Their efforts culminated in the meeting of the Cortes in 1810. Committees presented proposals for the delegates to consider. The Committee of Public Instruction presented a plan for a national system of education written by Gaspar Melchor de Jovellanos. Jovellanos, who had recommended tighter control of higher education during his brief tenure as secretary of grace and justice, now proposed uniform, compulsory, and free primary education, and the complete separation of arts and sciences in university instruction.[18]

For the liberal members of the Cortes, further reform from above was no longer sufficient. Rather, they endeavored to create a new kind of state in which power came from the people, and reform did not depend upon the whim of a monarch. For two long years the Cortes labored to write Spain's first written constitution. The result of their efforts was the Constitution of 1812, an exceedingly liberal document. After declaring that sovereignty rested in the Cortes itself, the document established a constitutional monarchy, turned subjects into citizens, abolished most of the traditional fueros, and guaranteed individual rights. The liberal Cortes, however, like the afrancesados in Madrid, represented only a small minority of the people. The nation applauded the delegates' patriotism far more enthusiastically than their liberalism. In truth, the liberal sitting in the Cortes and the afrancesado minister in Madrid may well have had more in common with each other than either had with the mass of the Spanish people.

Meanwhile, the Cortes initiated many changes in the structure of government. On July 27, 1811, it reunited the branches of medicine by reestablishing the Protomedicato. It endowed the Protomedicato with the same all-encompassing jurisdiction as it had possessed in 1780, but provided that its membership consist of two physicians, two surgeons, and one pharmacist. Medicine and surgery were to be equal in fact as well as in theory. However, the Cortes reserved for itself the right to initiate further reforms in education, hospital care, licensing procedures, and public health regulations.[19] Thus, within a period of six months both the Cortes and the Napoleonic government reunited medicine and centralized all education.

While the Cortes was deliberating in Cádiz and Joseph Napoleon

18. See Artola, *Los orígenes*, I, 265–271.

19. AHN, Consejos, Colección de Reales Cédulas, No. 1913, Decreto del Consejo de Regencia, July 27, 1811.

was initiating reforms in Madrid, Spanish and British forces gradually pressed toward the Spanish capital. In August 1812 the allied forces triumphantly entered Madrid. The French returned briefly a few months later, but on May 22, 1813, Joseph Napoleon withdrew for the last time. The Cortes and its executive arm, the Council of Regency, moved to Madrid. Unaware that Ferdinand VII would suppress all of its reforms, the Cortes set out to establish a new liberal regime in all Spain.

The College of San Carlos did not actively participate in the Cortes government either before or after the French withdrawal. In 1810 the college had ignored a request for its able-bodied instructors and students to join the patriot army.[20] Between the departure of Joseph and the return of Ferdinand VII, the school seemingly endeavored to remain as inconspicuous as possible. The Cortes did not appoint any surgeons associated with San Carlos to the restored Protomedicato, although José Ribes, a San Carlos professor, was elected to the Cortes by a Madrid constituency.[21]

San Carlos received official notification of the restoration of the Protomedicato on September 30, 1812. That restored body would supervise the school until Ferdinand regained his throne in February 1812. The interim government treated the Madrid surgeons remarkably well, considering that they had collaborated with the French and had declined to assist the patriot cause. All faculty members retained their positions. The Protomedicato endeavored to assist the school in solving its financial difficulties.[22] Indeed, the only sign of vengeance was a decree that invalidated all licenses granted during the French occupation. Holders of such licenses had to pay all fees again in order to be certified. The Protomedicato also took a step backward by restoring the licensing procedures in effect in 1780. Once again formal training was unnecessary for a license to practice surgery.[23]

The medical posture of the Cortes government was contradictory. On one hand, it planned government colleges oriented toward the natural sciences. The Protomedicato took steps to vaccinate all citizens.[24] It unified the faculties. On the other hand, it restored an institu-

20. AFM, Libro de Representactiones, Ordenes, etc., Orden del Conde de Cabarrías, Feb. 26, 1810.

21. AUC, Libro de Acuerdos (1810–1816), Junta of Sept. 2, 1816.

22. AUC, Libro de Ordenes, Oficio of Sept. 22, 1812; Libro de Acuerdos (1810–1816), Juntas of July 19, Oct. 28, Nov. 11, 1813; Jan. 2, 1814. All professors were to receive half salary until licensing exams replenished the treasury.

23. AUC, Libro de Ordenes, Oficio of June 18, 1813.

24. AUC, Libro de Acuerdos (1810–1816), Junta of July 19, 1813.

tion associated with the superiority of the physician and returned the surgeon to his former condition as a craftsman, not a professional scientist. The arrangement, of course, was temporary, but the patriot physicians could not resist the temptation to restrict the self-righteous surgeons who had even collaborated with the enemy to maintain their status. Perhaps the colleges of surgery were simply too closely associated with the hated Godoy and the French invaders. Or perhaps the Cortes felt that the requirements for surgery must be kept as simple as possible in order to open the profession to as many as possible and alleviate the terrible shortage of surgeons existing in Spain. Whatever the case, neither the reforms of the Cortes nor those of Joseph Napoleon would long endure. They served only to illustrate the thinking of both liberal factions and to provide models for later generations of reformers.

Ferdinand VII reentered Spain in March 1814. Two months later, assured of considerable support from his subjects, he nullified the constitution and restored all political institutions to their status before the 1808 invasion. For the next six years he ruled Spain arbitrarily and unimaginatively. Vengeful toward afrancesado and Cortes liberal alike, he tried in vain to return Spain to the days of absolutism, before liberals and reformers had begun tampering with tradition and the status quo. Ferdinand feared new ideas and was hostile toward education. Meanwhile, liberals began conspiring to overthrow the monarch and restore the constitution. The result was greater repression. In 1815 the Crown established a system of classifying prominent individuals according to their politics.

During the years following Ferdinand's return, Spanish education fell victim to the inefficiency, virtual bankruptcy, and closemindedness of the restored regime. Of necessity, Ferdinand replaced efficient administrators with those who had supported his 1808 and 1814 coups. Government finances were in disastrous shape, forcing severe retrenchment where politically feasible. Government salaries were in arrears; revenue from taxes, which amounted to less than half that of the years preceding 1808, could not come near meeting expenses. Spain herself was entering a long period of economic decline. Despite feeble efforts at reform, the Crown displayed far more enthusiasm in rooting out whatever liberalism remained in the nation's institutions of higher education. As a result, higher education had to fight for its very survival.[25]

25. On the reign of Ferdinand VII, see esp. Federico Suárez, "Fernando VII" *Estudios Americanos*, IV (1952), 5–25; Charles Wentz Fehrenbach, "Moderados and

The best example of the effect of Crown policy toward education was the fate of the University of Salamanca. For half a century its faculty had been engaged in modernizing the curriculum and opening its doors to new ideas. In early 1814 liberal professors presented the Cortes with a broad outline of a national, uniform system of education based upon the sciences from the primary grades through the university. Useful subjects would replace theology and canons once and for all. The university would truly respond to national needs.[26]

Ferdinand VII saw the needs of the nation differently. In early 1815 his council observed that some professors at Salamanca and other schools had promoted viewpoints that were "destructive to religion and conducive to the subversion of legitimate authority." In order to weed out the malefactors, the council appointed a commission to investigate each of the offensive institutions, remove the guilty professors, and replace dangerous texts with those that contained "wholesome doctrines."[27] At the same time the Crown created a board to draw up a new plan of studies for all Spanish universities.[28] As the fiscal of the council observed, education should contribute not only to national welfare but also to "the security of the state."[29]

The report of the commission that visited Salamanca emphasized the unsalutary effects of the years of curriculum revision. It recommended that the school return to the textbooks enumerated in the 1771 plan of studies with the proviso that every teacher lecture only on the doctrines contained in those texts.[30] Meanwhile, the recalcitrant University of Alcalá with the council's approval returned to the 1771 plan.[31]

In October 1817 the Crown ordered all universities to readopt the

---

Exaltados: The Liberal Opposition to Ferdinand VII, 1814–1832," *Hispanic American Historical Review*, L (1970), 55–56; Josep Fontana Lazaro, *La quiebra de la monarquía absoluta, 1814–1820* (Barcelona, 1971), pp. 47–57.

According to Fontana Lazaro, annual government revenue fell from an average of 1,439 million reales between 1798 and 1807 to only 658 million between 1814 and 1819. It climbed only a little (to 838 million) between 1824 and 1833.

26. AHN, Consejos, Leg. 5468, Parte 1, Exp. 58, Plan de Estudios y de instrucción pública presentado a las Cortes ordinarias por la Universidad de Salamanca, 1814.

27. AHN, Consejos, Leg. 5445, Expediente . . . en que se nombra Visitadores de los Estudios Reales, Acuerdo del Consejo, Feb. 6, 1815.

28. AHN, Consejos, Leg. 5496, Real Cédula, March 21, 1815.

29. AHN, Consejos, Leg. 5445, Expediente . . . en que se nombra Visitadores de los Estudios Reales, Informe del Fiscal, Feb. 24, 1815.

30. AHN, Consejos, Leg. 5468, Parte 1, Exp. 58, Informe sobre la Visita de la Universidad de Salamanca, 1815.

31. AHN, Universidades, Sig. 1232, Testimonio del Rector Francisco Gerónimo, Jan. 14, 1817.

1771 plan of studies, including its texts, degree requirements, and distribution of chairs. Only medicine would continue according to the 1804 revision.[32] The conservatives were finally victorious. The 1771 plan, conceived in its day as a first step of more substantial reform, was imposed as a reaction to all the progress that had come about since its creation.

The College of San Carlos also suffered a decline after the return of Ferdinand VII. In August 1814 the monarch inspected the school and was reportedly fascinated by the collection of surgical instruments. Unfortunately, his personal fascination did not deter him from suppressing the reunited Protomedicato and reestablishing the three separate administrative boards as they had existed in 1808. In November the king replaced Antonio Gimbernat and his colleagues on the Superior Board of Surgery with his own appointees.[33]

Gimbernat was now eighty-three years of age and almost blind. His illustrious career had contributed much to Spanish surgical education, but his dedication to San Carlos and to surgery regardless of contemporary politics earned him nothing but hardship in his final years. As a result of the system of political classification he lost his pension. In a pathetic letter he begged the Crown to provide him with some subsistence to alleviate his "most painful and deplorable situation." The Crown consented, but refused to continue the pension for his son, as was customary. Antonio Gimbernat died in November 1816, seemingly unappreciated except by his former colleagues at San Carlos. The school he had founded commemorated his death with public lectures and commissioned a marble bust in his memory.[34]

The death of Antonio Gimbernat marked the end of San Carlos' predominant position in Spanish medicine. San Carlos, like the university during the reign of Charles IV, became the recipient, not the instigator, of new plans of study. All but one member of the faculty at San Carlos in 1816 had come there after 1800. The school continued to fulfill its obligation to educate future surgeons, but San Carlos had become just another school, its prestige and influence a thing of the past.

The records of San Carlos suggest that the political repression fol-

32. AHN, Consejos, Leg. 5438, Expediente . . . por la que . . . quiese S.M. que se observe . . . el modo . . . antes del plan de 1807, Orden del Consejo, Oct. 29, 1817.

33. AUC, Libro de Acuerdos (1810–1816), Junta of Aug. 17, 1814; Libro de Ordenes, Oficios of Sept. 17, Nov. 16, 1814.

34. ARP, Sección de Empleados, Expediente de Antonio Gimbernat; AUC, Libro de Acuerdos (1810–1816), Junta of Nov. 16, 1816.

lowing Ferdinand's return only mildly inconvenienced the school. The new Superior Board repeatedly demanded that the college submit all its records, including minutes of faculty meetings, to government inspection. Presumably, the government was eager to find out how much the faculty had collaborated with the French. Whatever the reason, the junta consistently refused to comply. It maintained possession of its own archives, even when José Ribes, a vice director, was temporarily suspended for disobeying orders. At least one professor, Sebastián Loche, publicly defended his service to the French by arguing that what was good for surgery was ultimately good for the Spanish people, regardless of politics. His political classification cost him his chair.[35]

Meanwhile, the traditional cooperation between the college and the Superior Board all but disappeared. The board gave the Hospital General permission to train surgeons on its own, despite advice to the contrary from San Carlos. On several occasions the board demanded that a student receive a license when the San Carlos faculty believed the candidate was not sufficiently prepared to practice surgery. Sometimes the board even turned down the school's nominations for resident students and made its own selections. In 1815 the professors of San Carlos unanimously adopted a motion that censured the board for its "arbitrary orders using repugnant language."[36]

The Superior Board, for its part, had good reason for treating the school harshly. The once high standards of San Carlos were falling dramatically. Professors and students alike missed classes all too frequently. The renowned Thursday assemblies occurred only sporadically. Serious disciplinary problems illustrated a discouraging lack of dedication on the part of the students. Some mischievous students began dropping pieces of skeletons in the streets near the college, to the consternation of the civil authorities. The standards for certification also declined as some romance surgeons managed to bluff their way through examinations without even an elementary understanding of anatomy and surgery. Even the reputation of the school suffered. When Rafael Costa lost a patient, the faculty felt obligated to publish an explanation.

Indeed, medicine itself seemed to be declining. The number of Latin

35. AUC, Libro de Acuerdos (1810–1816), Juntas of Sept. 1, Oct. 5, Oct. 12, 1815; Aug. 19, 1816.

36. *Ibid.*, Juntas of Feb. 8, 1816; Jan. 30, Oct. 17, Nov. 20, 1817; June 11, June 18, 1818; AUC, Libro de Ordenes, Oficio of Sept. 28, 1815.

students remained small. In 1818, for example, San Carlos graduated some 130 romance students but only nine Latin students.[37] The same was true in Spain as a whole. According to one estimate, all but *fifty* of the more than two hundred surgeons practicing in Madrid were romance surgeons with no formal education.[38] So many surgeons in rural Spain had somehow procured licenses with no education that the Superior Board ordered all future applicants for licenses to present their books and instruments to the examining board as evidence of their serious study.[39] Meanwhile, as indicative of continuing prejudice against surgery, an anonymous bureaucrat listed the names of physicians with the respectful prefix "Don," but he did not do the same for surgeons.[40]

Since 1814, opposition to Ferdinand's harsh rule, particularly among the middle class and young army officers, had been growing. Conspiracies and periodically attempted coups increased the Crown's preoccupation with security matters. Frustrated liberals finally saw their opportunity when, on January 1, 1820, Colonel Rafael Riego initiated a coup in Cádiz among soldiers preparing for duty in America. Successful conspiracies followed in other cities. In March Ferdinand promised to obey the Constitution of 1812 and allowed the formation of a liberal junta in Madrid. The Cortes reconvened in July, and the king himself became a virtual prisoner of the new regime that called itself a constitutional monarchy. For the next three years the liberals of the War of Independence had another opportunity to try to rule Spain. Unfortunately, serious divisions within the ranks of the liberals themselves hampered their effectiveness. The moderately liberal Cortes, which ruled in Madrid until the summer of 1822, managed to institute substantial reforms, but the radical Cortes that succeeded it created so much chaos that almost nothing went into effect.

For Spain as a whole the liberal interlude was a time of political turmoil that saw the abolition of many traditional institutions and practices. For San Carlos it was a time of frequent governmental inspections, rapid changes in its legal position, and restoration of its reformist

37. AUC, Libro Tercera de Reválides (1816–1820).

38. AHN, Consejos, Leg. 3514, Exp. 17, Parte 1, Representación de la Junta Superior Gobernativa de Cirugía al Secretario de Estado y del Despacho de Gracia y Justicia, Dec. 10, 1816.

39. AUC, Libro de Ordenes, Oficio of June 15, 1818.

40. AGS, Dir. Gral. del Tesoro, Inventario 24, Leg. 977, Noticias de la Junta Superior Gobernativa de Cirugía a la Dirección General, July 1–Dec. 31, 1818.

zeal. Through it all the college managed to hold classes and carry on examinations without interruption. Only the Thursday assemblies were frequently postponed.

Once in power, the liberals immediately set to work completing the reforms of 1812. Uniformity and centralization were their keynotes. The Cortes quickly suppressed the separate administrative boards and again restored the Protomedicato, granting it authority over all education and licensing.[41] However, the very concept of the law treating men of medicine as special cases was under attack, as were many other traditional fueros. A committee of the Cortes proposed a board of health that would include not only physicians and surgeons but also lawyers, chemists, and economists.[42] Even San Carlos protested the legal autonomy of the traditional Protomedicato.

Meanwhile, every branch of government eagerly began collecting information from which it hoped to bring rational, orderly reform to Spain. San Carlos received requests for information from the Protomedicato, various committees of the Cortes, the Ministry of the Interior, and the provincial and city governments of Madrid. After 1821 San Carlos had to submit quarterly reports on class enrollment, examination results, and finances. In addition to information, the governmental bodies were also interested in proposals for reforming the college. The faculty was happy to oblige and spent much of the next few years reevaluating every aspect of the curriculum. The beleaguered secretary of the college begged the college for money to hire an assistant.[43]

On June 29, 1821, the Cortes approved a new master plan for all of Spanish education. It placed all schools under the jurisdiction of a General Office of Education (*Dirección General de Estudios.*) For San Carlos this meant that its direction switched from the medical profession itself back to the overseers of all educational establishments. The new Office of Education immediately reunited San Carlos and the Royal School of Practical Medicine, dubbing the combined institution the Special School for the Science of Healing. The enlarged faculty set to work drawing up a revised curriculum for the new school. Once again there was to be no distinction between physician and surgeon.

41. AUC, Libro de Ordenes, Oficio of Aug. 21, 1820; Copiador de Reales Ordenes (1818–1829), Real orden, Oct. 12, 1820.

42. Ley Orgánica de Sanidad Pública de la Monarquía Española, June 20, 1820. Mss. is in the Academia de Medicina.

43. AUC, Libro de Ordenes, Oficio of Oct. 28, 1822. His request was granted. On the surveys themselves, see AUC, Libro de Acuerdos (1817–1821), Juntas of May 25, July 30, Oct. 5, 1820; April 12, Aug. 31, 1821.

The master plan also enacted the long-forgotten dream of the Conde de Aranda to establish in Madrid a modern national university dedicated to the sciences. The Cortes moved the remaining faculties of Alcalá to Madrid, established new chairs in the sciences, including those of mechanics, mineralogy, and agronomy, and attached several academies in Madrid to the new institution. This new Central University was to set the pace for all Spanish higher education. The existing universities lost all their autonomy as they, too, fell under the immediate supervision of the General Office of Education.[44]

The most important accomplishment, however, was not the centralized educational structure itself but the establishment of two far more basic principles for all education. Both were the logical result of the liberal effort to abolish all traditional fueros and establish genuine equality among all citizens.

In late 1820 the Cortes abolished all requirements of purity of blood. Henceforth, all Spanish citizens were eligible to apply for any position in Spain regardless of blood or former convictions of their ancestry. There would be no more artificial distinctions between one man and another. At the same time the Cortes endeavored to make this ideal of equality a fact by establishing the principle that money would no longer be a barrier to obtaining an education or entering a profession. It established a maximum fee of 1,500 reales for any medical license. The 1822 regulations reaffirmed the principle by forbidding any national school from charging any tuition or fee except for a nominal matriculation fee.[45]

Liberal reform came to a temporary halt in April 1823 when French troops abruptly invaded the country and restored the authority of Ferdinand VII. That monarch, having learned nothing from the liberal intervention, was determined to turn the clock back to 1820. This time the reactionary king showed his opponents little mercy. There was no doubt in his mind that the participants in the Cortes government were revolutionaries and traitors. One indication of the temper of the times was the new form of request for critiques of medical works. The San Carlos professors were to report not only on the scientific accuracy

44. AUC, Copiador de Reales Ordenes, (1818–1829), Real orden, Sept. 18, 1821; Libro de Ordenes, Oficios of Sept. 25, Sept. 28, Oct. 9, Dec. 11, 1821. For the effects of the new regulations on the universities see La Fuente, *Historia de las universidades*, IV, 364–370.

45. AUC, Copiador de Reales Ordenes (1818–1829), Reales órdenes, Nov. 12, Dec. 13, 1820; Libro de Ordenes, Oficio of Aug. 23, 1822. The surgical colleges charged a matriculation fee of twenty-five reales, which was sent to the General Office of Education. The government supplied all operating funds.

of a book but also on its conformity to "the principles of our Sacred Religion and the Royal Privileges" of the king.[46]

During the months following the victory over liberalism, the Crown moved rapidly to revoke every action of the Cortes. A royal decree reestablished the three autonomous superior administrative boards and separated the School of Practical Medicine from San Carlos.[47] University reform was similarly undone. In rapid succession the Crown suppressed the Central University in Madrid, reestablished Alcalá, and imposed a curriculum that was "completely monarchical and Christian." Although the new plan introduced new courses and texts to the study of medicine, the classroom lectures remained isolated from practical application in the clinic.[48]

There was little doubt as to where the San Carlos faculty's sympathies lay. In 1820 every member eagerly took an oath of allegiance to the constitutional regime. More recently, the institution had allowed students to join the liberal forces fighting the French without losing course credits, and it had exempted all members of the constitutional militia from paying fees. Such exceptions were necessary, the professors had agreed, to preserve the nation from "a most ferocious despotism."[49] Now the despot was on the throne. Although the professors expected some setbacks, such as the separation of the faculties, the "ferocity" of the repression must have come as a surprise.

San Carlos had survived political turmoil in the past, but this time individuals were penalized simply for learning and teaching medicine during the rebel regime. The profession itself became the monopoly of those who were consistently and overtly loyal to Ferdinand VII. Only a critical personal illness convinced the monarch that the efficacy of medicine does not depend upon the politics of the practitioner.

The Crown first moved to dismiss all personnel overtly associated with liberalism. On July 4 the government demanded the dismissal of all professors who had not been on the faculty in 1820. Hesitancy on the part of the junta brought an angry ultimatum from the Superior Board. The junta still refused to dismiss the three professors involved,

46. For example, AUC, Libro de Acuerdos (1823–1827), Junta of Feb. 10, 1825.

47. AUC, Copiador de Reales Ordenes (1818–1829), Real orden, June 15, 1823.

48. AHN, Universidades, Sig. 1232, *Real Cédula de S.M. y Señores del Consejo, en la cual se fijan las reglas que han de observarse para que se restituya a las Universidades y demás Establecimientos Literarios del Reino la sana enseñanza; y para el abono o inadmisión de los cursos ganados y Grados conferidos en ellas en la época del titulado Gobierno Constitucional* (Madrid, 1824), July 21, 1824.

49. ACC, Libro de Acuerdos (1817–1821), Junta of March 29, 1820; Libro de Acuerdos (1823–1827), Juntas of Jan. 17, March 5, March 8, 1823.

arguing that they had won their position by oposición, not by mere appointment. Eventually the Crown relented and allowed them to stay. Meanwhile, it demanded a list of activities of all the other professors during the liberal regime. Anyone who had participated in the tribunals or militia of the Cortes government, or who had taken part in rioting, was also subject to dismissal. The government agents must have been efficient, for despite the reticence of the faculty, the Crown singled out two laboratory employees who were immediately fired.[50]

Ferdinand VII was not content to rely on personal confessions and informers to weed out all those who had collaborated with liberalism. On July 1 a royal cédula created military tribunals before which every government employee had to "purify himself" in order to retain his position.[51] Thus, the burden of proof fell on the individual. It would have been virtually impossible for the San Carlos professors to prove their innocence, as they had, in fact, cooperated with the Cortes. Although the professors retained their chairs, the uncertainty of their future remained unresolved for two years.

Students of San Carlos during the liberal regime also were victims of the royal vengeance. In February 1824 the Crown annulled all licenses granted during the reign of "the revolutionary system." The royal order explained that this step was to protect the public, since education had become so decadent under liberalism. Moreover, recipients of the illegitimate licenses had neither submitted proof of their baptism and purity of blood nor paid the fees required by the statutes. Future candidates for certification would have to document the purity of their political behavior during the rebellion. According to a decree the following July, such documentation was necessary merely to matriculate at any school.[52] How strictly these restrictions were enforced is, however, an open question.

The application of loyalty tests to students may have been the result of the considerable student dissension that occurred during these years. According to the educational historian Vicente de la Fuente, a contemporary, by the 1820s some students were becoming political activists.[53] The San Carlos records bear out this claim. Frequent requests from the

50. AUC, Libro de Acuerdos (1823–1827), Juntas of July 11, Sept. 4, Sept. 17, 1823; Copiador de Reales Ordenes (1818–1829), Real orden, Aug. 9, 1823. One of the three professors under attack was Juan Castelló, son of the reformer Pedro Castelló.

51. AUC, Libro de Acuerdos (1823–1827), Junta of Oct. 29, 1823.

52. AUC, Copiador de Reales Ordenes (1818–1829), Real orden, Feb. 10, 1824; Libro de Ordenes, Oficio of Oct. 7, 1824.

53. La Fuente, *Historia de las universidades*, IV, 372, 385.

Superior Board for information on the "political behavior" of specific students and a prohibition against students bearing arms plainly indicate what was going on. The San Carlos junta justified holding all classes in the morning by noting that if students left the building after dark they were likely to create incidents involving the French soldiers on guard duty nearby.

A remarkable series of events brought the persecution of the school to an end. In early 1825 Ferdinand suffered an acute attack of the gout that had plagued him most of his life. He called Pedro Castelló, a professor at San Carlos who had delivered one of his children, to attend him. After weeks of constant care, the monarch recovered. Apparently his experience made the king more sympathetic toward the requests of Castelló.[54] At any rate, during 1825 all the San Carlos professors and many of its graduates appeared before the military tribunal and readily received their certificates of purification. Castelló himself received an appointment to the Superior Administrative Board.[55] His personal influence on the king was limitless.

Pedro Castelló's laudatory biographer may have exaggerated his role in the rapid "purification" of San Carlos faculty. Ferdinand VII, who always had enemies on the right as well as the left, was not a complete opponent of progress. He consistently persecuted Spanish universities and colleges in order to repress liberalism, but he could be sympathetic to the nonpolitical sciences.

In any case, in 1827 the Crown reunited medicine and surgery and approved a new curriculum for San Carlos.[56] Its author was Pedro Castelló. He had first written the new regulations in 1822 in response to an order from the Cortes to modernize medical education. A combination of happy circumstances had restored liberalism to medical education.

Liberals regained power after the death of Ferdinand VII in 1833. During the long reign of his daughter Isabel II, a succession of liberal ministries hesitatingly moved Spain toward representative government. Although the conservative revolt of the Carlists compounded the disagreement among the liberals themselves, there was a general feeling

54. Eusebio Castelo Serra, *Biografía del Cirujano-Médico Pedro Castelló, Marqués de la Salud* (Madrid, 1850). Castelló had fled from Madrid in 1809 rather than collaborate with the French.

55. AUC, Copiador de Reales Ordenes (1818–1829), Reales órdenes, June 26, July 23, Aug. 12, Aug. 17, Sept. 27, Oct. 3, 1825.

56. ARP, Leg. 691, Reglamento científico, económico e interior de los Reales Colegios de Medicina y Cirugía, y de los Profesores que ejerzan estas facultades, June 30, 1827. The regulations were published in a royal cédula the following year.

in Madrid that such eighteenth-century goals as uniformity, central control, and progress should be the basis of government policy.

Higher education remained an important element in the liberal efforts to modernize Spain. Although the specific educational programs enacted under Isabel II are beyond the scope of this study, their broad objectives were not unlike those of Antonio Gimbernat and the advisers to Charles III. Ironically, their fulfillment led to the suppression of San Carlos itself.

The debate over medical education never completely subsided during the tumultuous years that followed Napoleon's invasion. After 1820 unification of the medical faculties became a public issue, argued in pamphlets and periodicals. Thoughtful arguments were presented on both sides. Unfortunately, however, many medical reformers became so embroiled in the unification issue that they tended to overlook such more basic questions as the purpose and content of medical education itself. Indeed, all of Spanish education suffered during the first half of the nineteenth century as disputes over jurisdiction and privilege overshadowed those of curriculum and teaching methods.[57]

While some physicians and surgeons debated the legal issues, others turned to philosophy and history. In a trend that has continued down to the present, they took to analyzing the epistemological implications of clinical procedures and writing histories of their own professions. In a society that valued intellectuals and artists over scientists, the doctor became an intellectual and an artist. Antonio Hernández Morejón, a San Carlos professor during the 1820s, exemplified this trend.[58]

In any case, the advocates of a unified profession achieved a victory when in 1828 the Crown promulgated the regulations drawn up by Pedro Castelló. Once again all schools, including university medical faculties, would follow a single broad curriculum that encompassed internal and external medicine alike. Professors would specialize in one area of medicine and would not rotate from one chair to another. Other royal decrees united the two faculties in the Royal Palace, including the honorary positions, and in the armed forces.[59]

In writing his statutes, Castelló realized that no simple reorganizing

57. Galli, *Contestación al informe*, was indicative of the debate. The pamphlet includes long quotations from advocates and opponents of unification.

58. His *Historia bibliográfica de la medicina española*, still valuable, and *Ensayo de ideología clínica* (Madrid, 1821), are good examples of this trend. Hernández Morejón also edited the *Décadas médico-quirúrgicas y farmacéuticas*, a journal that opened its pages to the debates that embroiled the profession.

59. ARP, Leg. 689, Real decreto relativo al arreglo de Facultativos de Medicina y Cirugía de la Real Cámara y Familia, Sept. 7, 1827.

of the school system could immediately supply Spain with all the practitioners it needed. Accordingly, he, too, decided he had to compromise his high standards by allowing semitrained practitioners in rural areas. The surgeon-bleeder (*cirujano-sangrador*), as he was called, would take an abbreviated three-year course, after which he would be qualified to perform simple surgical procedures, deliver babies, and provide simple remedies. The surgeon-bleeder remained a fixture in Spain well into the second half of the century.

In 1834 the long years of perseverence under trying physical conditions at San Carlos were finally rewarded. The school moved to a newly constructed building especially designed for the college near the Hospital of the Passion.[60] None of the school's founders lived to see the quarters that Charles III had first promised in 1785.

Meanwhile, with the restoration of liberalism in 1833, every aspect of the medical establishment was again publicly debated. The issues were familiar—the unity of the faculties, the existence of several classes of practitioners, and the role of university medical faculties. (For political reasons the Crown had temporarily suppressed the universities in 1830). Years of arbitrary reorganizations had created distrust and bitterness on both sides. Yet the articles and letters to the editor in the medical press were reminiscent of the memoranda sent to the Council of Castile during the reign of Charles III.

Most writers agreed that unification was correct. They looked back with disgust at the petty competition between the separate juntas and noted that medicine and surgery were no longer separate anywhere in Europe. However, there was far less unanimity in support of a national system of medical schools following a standardized curriculum drawn up in Madrid. Proponents of uniformity argued that national standards would raise the level of education everywhere and noted the success of uniformity abroad. Opponents answered that diversity would lead to greater innovations.[61]

Underlying the opposition to a national system of medical education were the years of outside interference suffered by the universities.

60. AUC, Libro de Acuerdos (1830–1834), Junta of Oct. 10, 1834.

61. Pedro Castelló, *Memoria sobre el arreglo de la Ciencia de Curar que presentó a la Dirección General de Estudios del Reino* (Madrid, 1836), pp. 7–18; "Funestes efectos del mal gobierno que ha tenido la Facultad hasta el presente," *Boletín de Medicina, Cirugía, y Farmacia* (hereinafter cited as *Boletín de Medicina*), II (1835), 437–440; Melchor Sánchez de Toca, *Memoria sobre el Plan de Estudios, la Organización y el Personal de la Escuelas Médicas Estranjeras con aplicaciones a la nacional de San Carlos de Madrid* (Madrid, 1840), pp. 1–5. These and the pamphlets cited below are preserved in the Academia de Medicina de Madrid.

University professors blamed the surgical schools for the decline of university medicine since those schools had monopolized the limited government financial support of education. Echoing the age-old disdain of the "craft" of surgery, they argued that the ability to think clearly and logically was more valuable to a doctor than was an impressive technique with the scalpel. They claimed that the founders of San Carlos had deliberately set out to blacken the reputation of university medicine, hoping to eventually destroy it, as evidenced by the suppression of their medical faculties in 1799.[62]

The liberals in power, on the other hand, had little sympathy for the universities and their glorious tradition. They hoped to replace that autonomous symbol of privilege and backwardness with a national system of education. Henceforth, a central authority would set the standards and draw up the curricula for every school in Spain. Education was too important to entrust entirely to the educators, who were too often more interested in their own welfare than in that of the nation. The school, like every other institution, had to be subordinate to the needs of the state. Such policies soon destroyed the separate identity not only of the universities but also of San Carlos.

The final efforts toward complete standardization of all higher education began in 1835 with the appointment of a commission of professors and administrators to draw up a model curriculum.[63] Pedro Castelló was a member.[64] After eight years of hard work, the commission recommended the suppression of every school and faculty of medicine. Two categories of uniform national facilities would replace faculties and colleges. The faculty, which would be established in principal cities, would provide a complete course in medicine and surgery. The recommended seven-year plan of studies included preliminary classes in the natural sciences and three years of clinical training. Castelló presumably intended that San Carlos would become the faculty of medicine in Madrid. The college, on the other hand, would offer a shorter course to train men in minor surgery, elementary medicine, and obstetrics.[65]

62. José Corenzo Pérez and Manuel Hermenegildo Davila, *Observaciones sobre el Nuevo Plan de Estudios Médicos* (Madrid, 1844), pp. 3–20; "Defensa de la instrucción médica en las universidades," *Boletín de Medicina*, II (1835), 123–126; Letter from "L. A.," *Boletín de Medicina*, II (1835), 141–142.

63. "Real decreto," Nov. 1, 1835, in *Boletín de Medicina*, II (1835), 441.

64. *Instrucciones generales sobre el orden y método de enseñanza en las Facultades Médicas del Reino* (Madrid, 1846).

65. Plan de Estudios Médicos, 1843, quoted in part in García del Real, *Historia de la Medicina en España*, pp. 609 ff.

Meanwhile, the reestablished General Office of Education tackled the reorganization of higher education as a whole. The result of its efforts was the creation of a system of national universities under the direct supervision of a Ministry of Public Instruction.[66] The curricula of specific faculties would be identical everywhere. At the same time the Crown finally fulfilled the dream of Aranda back in the 1770s by creating a national university in Madrid.

The Literary University of Madrid formally opened its doors in October 1845. The principal speaker at the inaugural ceremonies described the new university as the fulfillment of the hopes of all "lovers of enlightenment and knowledge." Order would replace chaos, science would replace tradition. The faculty of medicine of the University of Madrid was the school that had once been known as the Royal College of San Carlos.[67]

To some extent the incorporation of San Carlos into the new University of Madrid fulfilled the goals of Gimbernat and his supporters. They, too, had fought for equality between medicine and surgery, for suppression of the more backward medical faculties, and for the progressive innovations adopted by San Carlos to become standard throughout Spain. In terms of legal structure and close government supervision, the regulations of 1845 accomplished more than the eighteenth-century reformers had dreamed possible.

Yet the academic excellence that had characterized San Carlos in its early years seems to have been a casualty of the Napoleonic invasion and the death of Antonio Gimbernat. As the junta struggled to cope with political demands, administrative reorganizations, and financial crises, little time remained for academic problems. A reading of the junta records after 1812 reveals little of the enthusiasm of earlier years.

In retrospect, no institution closely tied to government could have weathered the political chaos successfully. A succession of mediocre rulers, revolution and reaction, and changes for the sake of change so disrupted San Carlos and similar schools that success was eventually defined as simple existence. Once government deprived San Carlos of its voice in national policies, innovation seemed less important than careful adherence to edicts from above. In addition, the social prej-

66. *Plan de Estudios decretado por S.M. en 17 de septiembre de 1845* (Madrid, 1845).

67. Lorenzo Arrazola, *Discurso Inaugural pronunciado en la solemne apertura de la Universidad Literaria de Madrid* (Madrid, 1845).

udices that discouraged outstanding young men from studying surgery continued to plague the college. To be sure, the progressive curriculum outlined in the statutes remained. But the zeal of the reformer and the curiosity of the scholar seemed to decline with the retirement and death of its earlier faculty. After 1812 San Carlos was no longer the harbinger of modern medicine but simply a good school for studying surgery.

A cursory glance at the commentaries on Spanish medicine at mid-century were hauntingly reminiscent of the remarks of Father Feijóo, Martín Martínez, and others. Classroom instruction was still divorced from the laboratory and the clinic. Spanish schools still lagged behind those of other European nations. One critic bemoaned the fact that medical students from Spain's former colonies studied in every European country but Spain.[68] Financial support was never adequate. Bureaucratic red tape and institutional lethargy hindered the progressive doctor from doing his best.

Yet the failure of San Carlos and, indeed, the failure of the Spanish Enlightenment were not complete and cannot be attributed to their sponsors. Indeed, the minority of progressive men such as Pedro Castelló who followed in their footsteps testify to their success. But centralized power, even when "enlightened," cannot change the minds and habits of men overnight. And the chaos that followed 1808 cut short even the attempt.

68. Pedro González Velasco, *Rápida ojeada sobre la anatomía en España* (Madrid, 1856). For other criticisms and shortcomings, see Sánchez de Toca, *Memoria*, esp. p. 11; García del Real, *Historia de la Medicina en España*, pp. 595–608; Juan Ramón Zaragoza Rubira, "Los hospitales españoles en el primer tercio del siglo XIX," *Medicina Española*, LXVIII (1962), 149–158.

CHAPTER VIII

# SAN CARLOS, MEDICAL REFORM, AND THE ENLIGHTENMENT

The College of San Carlos, like the Spanish Enlightenment itself, came about as a result of the efforts of many individual reformers. Apolitical surgeons proposed the creation of a school that would substantially improve the manner in which surgeons learned their professions. The progressive advisers of Charles III accepted the proposal and used the new school to reform and restrict the universities and the Royal Protomedicato, the two institutions that had traditionally dominated Spanish medicine. During the reign of Charles IV the founders of San Carlos became royal counselors themselves. Using San Carlos as their model, they attempted to renovate all medical education according to their own design. In the process they became so closely identified with liberalism that after 1808 the very innovations they had advocated became political issues.

San Carlos was representative of the type of reform to which the Spanish ilustrado dedicated himself. Antonio Gimbernat, Mariano Rivas, Pedro Virgili, and Pedro Castelló were probably typical of countless Spaniards in schools, professions, and societies during the eighteenth century. Their family and academic backgrounds varied greatly. They came from all parts of Spain, although many of the surgical reformers were Catalan. Most were remarkably indifferent to broad questions of ideology and public policy.

The medical reformers were, above all, pragmatic. Gimbernat and his colleagues created a school specifically designed to train future surgeons in the precise skills they would need to practice successfully and thereby gain the respect of other practitioners. Courses and authors were chosen on their own merits; whether they were considered traditional or modern made no difference. Thus, assigned texts ranged from Hippocrates to Boerhaave and the reports of the Paris Academy of Surgery.

The efforts to improve surgery were not limited to academic matters. Within the realm of medicine Gimbernat was an astute observer. He realized that promising young men would not consider studying surgery until the profession itself earned public approbation and respect. Thus, he fought to remove surgery from the jurisdiction of the Protomedicato not only because that body allowed untrained men to become licensed surgeons but also because it treated the profession of surgery itself with age-long scorn and derision. Gimbernat's attitude toward Latin examinations and limpieza de sangre was similarly pragmatic. No manuscripts record his personal opinion on such traditional university practices, but he was determined to impose them on San Carlos so that its graduates would be held in the same high esteem as university graduates. Surgery was to become a liberal profession whose standards would surpass those of the more traditional careers.

The same practical approach characterized Gimbernat's attitude toward foreign ideas and practices. He was fully aware that Spanish medical education lagged behind the more advanced clinics and schools of England and France. Yet he was not so naïve as to believe that because a method was foreign it was automatically better. He deliberately selected such foreign practices as the clinic and the wax anatomical pieces, but he refused to impose any of the all-encompassing medical theories on San Carlos. His statutes instructed professors to be discriminating in their use of foreign books. Nevertheless, he frequently referred to foreign practices in order to bolster arguments for his own proposals.

In their complete dedication to improving Spanish surgery, the reformers were generally indifferent to political events. Seeing themselves as scientists, not statesmen, the San Carlos faculty attempted to carry on as usual in spite of the French occupation, the reaction under Ferdinand VII, and the liberal adventure of 1820. Indeed, the surgeons readily collaborated with any friend of surgery, be he Manuel de Godoy, Joseph Napoleon, or Ferdinand VII. Unfortunately such collaboration, plus the school's efforts to assert its influence over other institutions, led to medical education itself becoming a political issue in the squabbles between liberals and conservatives.

The principal obstacle the surgeons of San Carlos faced lay not in ministerial politics, however, but in the privileges and prerogatives of entrenched institutions, particularly the universities and the Protomedicato. The medical establishment, though cognizant of the need for change, was never willing to sacrifice its own prestige. San Carlos therefore represented a threat, not to old ideas, but to established standards of prestige and authority. As a result, its very existence made conflict inevitable.

Furthermore, the founders of San Carlos, themselves the victims of traditional prejudices, had little sympathy for those who disagreed with them. They were convinced that all innovation had to be patterned after San Carlos in order to be effective. They ignored the progressive members of the faculty of medicine at Salamanca, certain that the decadent university was beyond all hope. The same misunderstanding characterized the surgeons' relations with the Royal Protomedicato. Although that body was careless in its examinations and discriminatory toward surgeons, the Protomedicato was attempting to eliminate quackery while still providing Spain with as many surgeons as possible. Gimbernat and his colleagues, dedicated to training a small number of thoroughly competent practitioners, tended to ignore both the regulation of quackery and the severe shortage of any practitioners, fully trained or not. They also had little sympathy with the understandable desires of physicians and the Confradía de San Cosme y San Damian to maintain their traditional privileges.

The advisers of Charles III, particularly the Duque de Losada, had hesitated to give any single institution complete authority over an entire profession. Thus, the 1787 statutes of San Carlos had not deprived the recently reorganized Protomedicato of its licensing powers. When Gimbernat and his colleagues won a voice in government during the 1790s, however, they attempted to suppress all other institutional participation in the training and licensing of surgeons, and to impose their standards on medicine as well. To be sure, their reforms did succeed in further improving medical education. But had the monopoly of San Carlos and the Royal School of Practical Medicine been enforced, the shortage of trained practitioners would have become still worse. As it was, the united faculty of 1799 was responsible for delaying the establishment of a more modern medical curriculum at the University of Salamanca for at least five years.

Despite their later participation in government, there is no doubt that the ilustrados, at least in medicine, were indigenous to Spain, and not a mere by-product of the Bourbon dynasty. All received their education and training in Spanish institutions; many had even attended Spanish universities before the reforms of the 1770s. Moreover, both university reform and the new schools and academies were initiated by

Spanish physicians and surgeons—not by the Crown. The government of Charles III simply made their reforms a reality. Although committed to modernization, the Council of Castile proceeded slowly and deliberately, unwilling to accept change merely for the sake of change. Thus, it scrupulously solicited the opinion of all factions before taking any action. Before approving the proposals for the Madrid college the Council consulted individual physicians and surgeons, the Academy of Medicine, and the Protomedicato. (Curiously, it did not consult the universities, the very institutions then charged with training Latin surgeons.) Such thoroughness led to lengthy delays but avoided the type of impetuous change that occurred during the reign of Charles IV.

Although individuals outside of government initiated most academic reform, the Council of Castile and its hard-working fiscal, the Conde de Campomanes, frequently revised the proposals to conform with its own objectives. Before the reign of Charles III the Crown had generally accepted any promising proposal. Thus, the medical academies of Seville and Madrid and the surgical college of San Fernando had readily received royal approval. But it soon became clear that the plethora of new institutions was creating innumerable jurisdictional squabbles. New curricula could lead to widely divergent standards for degrees and licenses. Thus, Campomanes, though an ardent supporter of reform, also tried to bring order and uniformity into higher education. New university curricula had to conform to those of Salamanca. Similarly, the Duque de Losada recommended that the Protomedicato continue to license surgeons even if the applicant were educated at San Carlos. Soon after San Carlos opened, Gimbernat was encouraged to revise the statutes of the Barcelona college to conform with those of the school at Madrid. In that way the intervention of the Crown made uniformity and royal control almost as important as academic considerations in the reform of higher education.

Royal officials also gave careful attention to the cost of the new proposals they received. Since new schools and academies were expensive, they had to promise concrete results. Once they were established, the Crown exercised careful control over their budgets. In the case of San Carlos the Crown was most generous in its annual subsidy, but it still was reluctant to approve new programs that might prove costly. It recognized the value of clinics and public obstetrical instruction but delayed in granting final approval until sufficient funds could be found. Financial problems were presumably responsible for the endless delay in providing San Carlos with its own quarters. One of the principal arguments for granting San Carlos the right to license practitioners was that the examination fees would make the school self-supporting. Thus, it would appear that financial considerations, not fear of innovation, were often responsible for the hesitancy of the Crown to experiment.

The College of San Carlos itself was designed and operated by surgeons. It had no administrators from outside the profession. Surgeons drew up its ordinances, sat on its governing bodies, and administered its day-to-day activities. Since only experts made decisions on courses, faculty appointments, and examination requirements, San Carlos was able to maintain high professional standards. Unfortunately, the surgeons' hold on the school also forced it into the disputes between physicians and surgeons, making the college more controversial than it might have been. In addition, most members of the faculty in later years had once been students at one of the surgical colleges. Since the colleges represented the most progressive elements of the profession, such inbreeding was not initially harmful. However, the constant challenge of new ideas decreased in later years as the San Carlos faculty gained more confidence in the school. During the 1820s the minutes of the junta reveal less interest in foreign innovation and new techniques. The early enthusiasm for research and experiment seemed to disappear as the school became more self-satisfied.

In social terms San Carlos provided Spaniards of low birth with the opportunity to become respected professionals. Low fees, no tuition, and subsidies for resident students allowed young men with little money to become surgeons. At the same time the school's successful efforts to make its degrees equivalent to those of the universities enabled San Carlos graduates to enter the ranks of Spain's small middle class.

San Carlos contributed to the spirit of Enlightenment not only in its classroom but also by publicizing new knowledge and techniques to rural practitioners and to the lay public. Public disputations and anatomical demonstrations were popular in eighteenth-century Spain. By allowing auditors to attend its classes and lectures, San Carlos not only made new knowledge available but also contributed to bringing about a greater respect for observation and experiment, a major objective of the ilustrados. The weekly lectures and criticisms also provided the isolated rural surgeon with a ready source of expert advice. The censorship of medical books, though potentially harmful, safeguarded the public from the dangerous, erroneous ideas of medical practice that were all too prevalent.

The Madrid college also led to the downfall of the pernicious distinction between physicians and surgeons. The high standards, the progressive educational methods, and the imposition of such university requirements as purity of blood and fluency in Latin raised the public esteem of the surgeon. By 1800 San Carlos was clearly setting the standards for all medical education. Indeed, the college of surgeons eventually surpassed both the Royal Protomedicato and the medical faculties of universities in both prestige and influence. As a result, the surgeon himself became a respected member of the medical profession. No longer would he be the object of scorn and ridicule.

The paramount accomplishment of San Carlos, however, was in firmly establishing modern medicine and surgery in Spain. Although the education designed by Antonio Gimbernat contributed little that was completely new to the training of medical practitioners, it did effectively incorporate every major innovation of the eighteenth century. San Carlos then became the model for further reforms in medical education throughout Spain, assuming the role that Salamanca had played in the first phase of university reform. In addition, San Carlos did not simply introduce Spain to methods that were long in use elsewhere. Most medical schools throughout Europe still emphasized classical authors, philosophical speculation, and learning by rote. The schools that Gimbernat copied—the clinics of Leyden and Edinburgh, the classes of John Hunter—were not typical of medical education anywhere. Thus, Gimbernat created a model that was among the most progressive of any in Europe.

The San Carlos curriculum was novel for its day in both structure and content. Individual courses were based on logical divisions of surgery, not on specific authors. The material, not the author, became the basis of an education. The statutes of the college presupposed that the individual instructor would keep abreast of new knowledge and select the best text for his course. In addition, the San Carlos curriculum fortuitously prepared graduates to take advantage of the principal medical discoveries of the early nineteenth century. Anatomy, though much in vogue, had limited practical application in Gimbernat's lifetime. But when effective anesthetics and an understanding of germ theory made major surgery feasible, the San Carlos graduate had the knowledge of anatomy needed to operate. Gimbernat's insistence upon a strong background in the natural sciences was similarly fortunate as the application of biology and chemistry became increasingly important in modern medicine. Moreover, the San Carlos surgeons wisely ignored the popular quest for all-encompassing theories of life, a trend that rapidly became discredited.

Most important of all, San Carlos was in the forefront of the move of medicine from the classroom and individual sick room to the hospital clinic. Most medical reformers readily acknowledged that actual experience in treating illnesses must supplement the classroom lecture. Gimbernat also realized that such haphazard experience as apprentice surgeons received was still not sufficient. The student needed thorough, disciplined, practical experience under expert guidance on a large scale. In the San Carlos clinic the lessons were coordinated with explanatory lectures in the classrooms. The student learned orderly procedures of diagnosis and treatment. By coming in contact with many patients, the student learned to distinguish the signs common to a disease from those denoting complications. By following the progress of individual patients from the first diagnosis to the final cure, the student learned to evaluate the efficacy of specific treatments and medications. Through observation, comparison, experiment, and measurement the very practice of medicine became scientific. San Carlos introduced not only new knowledge and techniques but also an entirely new attitude toward surgical practice and research.

The Royal College of San Carlos succeeded in providing Spain with surgeons as well trained as any in Europe, and it provided a model for educational reforms elsewhere. However, its effect on Spanish medicine as a whole was not as great as its founders had originally hoped. To be sure, no single institution alone can reform an entire profession. In the case of San Carlos, though, the early enthusiasm and dedication of both the surgeons themselves and their supporters in government seemed to dissipate within one generation. When San Carlos became part of the University of Madrid, Spain still faced the basic problem of a severe shortage of trained doctors.

The shortcomings of Spanish science and technology are beyond the scope of this book. The history of San Carlos does, however, suggest possible explanations. Feijóo had blamed the lack of respect and interest in science for much of Spain's backwardness. Institutions such as San Carlos showed Spaniards the immense possibilities of science, but science itself never seemed to capture the imaginations of any large number of people. The constant political turmoil after 1808 made political activity appear to be a more immediate, effective means of improving Spanish life.

After 1808 government interest in the promotion of science and the useful arts also declined. Other programs took precedence in the competition for government financial support. Frequent insurrection and repression distracted government officials and made planning difficult. In addition, education itself became a political issue. Conservatives sought to use higher education to preserve orthodoxy and traditional values; liberals tried to create a centralized educational system to suppress university autonomy and backwardness. As a result, the Protomedicato, the proposal for a Madrid university, and the distinction between physicians and surgeons became symbols in ideological debates.

The surgeons of San Carlos were also responsible for the shortcomings of the school in the nineteenth century. The excellence of San Carlos in its early years was due to Gimbernat's total dedication to improving surgical education and research. He and his colleagues were surgeons, not political philosophers. They were more interested in setting up a clinic or discovering a new operating technique than in the juridical structure of Spanish education. They gave their complete attention to forming a curriculum, selecting texts, and establishing public anatomical demonstrations. A spirit of enthusiasm and innovation permeated the school as the faculty searched for new methods of instruction. Even the united faculty was created primarily for academic reasons.

Unfortunately, the very superiority of San Carlos led to the loss of its original enthusiasm and flexibility. The Superior Board became so infatuated with the success of the college that it set out to make it the model for all medical education in Spain. The institution that had been established to challenge traditional methods of education was slowly becoming as self-confident and set in its ways as the universities had been. Its faculty became increasingly conscious of honors and rank, and acted as if any school that differed from San Carlos was automatically inferior. The challenge of new types of teaching and research was replaced by the dream of administering a vast system of education.

Nevertheless, conflict between existing institutions and San Carlos was probably inevitable. The long struggle that had delayed the opening of the college convinced its surgeons that effective reforms were possible only if they had the authority to enforce them. Entrenched privileges, traditional biases, and institutional jealousies were not easily overcome. As a result, academic reform was necessarily a political matter, much as Gimbernat and his colleagues abhorred politics.

In sum, the controversy that permeated educational and scientific reform in eighteenth-century Spain was not primarily an intellectual one, at least not in medicine. Gimbernat and his colleagues seldom encountered significant opposition on academic grounds. Rather, the issue was one of jurisdiction and traditional autonomy. The enlightened surgeons of San Carlos realized that one school, no matter how progressive its curriculum, could not reform a profession. Hence, the ultimate success of San Carlos was not in its academics alone but in leading the way in reforming medical education everywhere. So, too, the failure of the Spanish Enlightenment to have a greater impact on Spain was not the result of ideas, either traditional or modern, but of the potency of existing institutions and the interests they represented to defend their prerogatives in the name of tradition.

# Bibliography of Works Used

## Manuscripts


Academia de Medicina de Madrid.

Actas de las Juntas de Gobierno del Real Colegio de Madrid durante los años 1795, 1796, 1797, y 1798.

Ley orgánica de sanidad pública de la monarquía española, 1820.

Varios papeles de estudios médicos, 1801.

Archivo de la Diputación Provincial de Madrid.

Serie Antiguo, Legajo 118.

Archivo de la Facultad de Medicina de la Universidad de Madrid.

Antiguo Colegio de San Carlos.

Juntas literarias.

Libro de Acuerdos, 1787–1804.

Libro de Acuerdos que se remitan a la Junta Superior para su aprobación antes de sentarlos en el libro, 1795–1800.

Libro de Cuentas: Entradas y salidas del caudal de dotación señalado al Real Colegio de San Carlos, 1786–1815.

Libro de representaciones, órdenes y repuestas, y reales cédulas, 1787–1817.

Lista de los médicos del Real Colegio de Medicina de Madrid que mandó establecer por S. M., 1796–1799.

Archivo de la Universidad Central.

Sección del Antiguo Colegio de San Carlos.

Copiador de Reales Ordenes, 1818–1829.

Libros de Acuerdos. 1804–1810, 1810–1816, 1817–1821, 1823–1827, 1828–1830, 1830–1834.

Libro de Contabilidad–Salidas de Caudales, 1791–1826.

Libro de Matrícula de Cirujanos Latinos, 1787–1817.

Libro de Matrículas de Romancistas, 1810–.

Libro de Matrículas Generales, 1801–1805.

Libro de Oposiciones–Cátedras, Vol. I.

Libro de órdenes y oficios comunicados por la Real Junta Superior Gobernativa de Cirugía al Real Colegio de San Carlos.

Libro Tercera de Reválidas, 1816–1820.

Registro de asuntos de la secretaría, 1802–1805.

Archivo del Real Palacio, Madrid.
Sección Administriva.
Legajos 689, 691.
Sección de Empleados.
Archivo General de Indias.
Sección de Gobierno, Indifferente General.
Legajo 1551.
Archivo General de Simancas.
Sección de Hacienda, Dirección General del Tesoro.
Inventario 24.
Legajo 977.
Sección de Hacienda, Secretaría.
Legajos 549, 952, 953.
Sección de Gracia y Justicia.
Legajos 404, 405 (Old Series 989, 990, 991).
Archivo Histórico Nacional.
Sección de Consejos.
Colección de Reales Cédulas, Núm. 606, 1036, 1913.
Legajos 511, 721, 783, 812, 924, 1035, 1285, 1845, 3514, 5430, 5436, 5438, 5444, 5445, 5459, 5460, 5462, 5464, 5465, 5467, 5468, 5469.
Libros de Gobierno 721e, 1349e, 1359e, 1368e.
Seccion de Universidades.
Legajo 42, 1175, 1232.
Signatura 1232.

## Selected Official Documents

*Below are listed printed and manuscript documents of special significance with their archival locations.*

Borrador de las Ordenanzas para el gobierno de los Hospitales General y Pasión de Madrid, 1747.
ADP, Leg. 118.

*Colección de reales decretos, órdenes y cédulas de su Magestad . . . dirigidas a está Universidad de Salamanca.* 3 vols. Salamanca, 1774.
AHN, Consejos, Leg. 5462, Exp. 39.

*Concordia y reales ordenanzas para el régimen y gobierno de la Facultad de Farmacia, formadas con conocimiento de la Real Junta General de Gobierno de la Facultad Reunida.* Madrid, 1800.
ARP, Sec. Administriva, Leg. 691.

*Constituciones y ordenanzas para el gobierno de los Reales Hospitales General, y de la Pasión de Madrid.* Madrid, 1760.
ADP, Leg. 118.

Consulta del Consejo de Castilla satisfaciendo a una Real Orden que expone

lo que se le ofrece esta facultad, y propone los medios que se podran adoptar a este fin, Aug. 23, 1774. (Cited as Consulta sobre cirugía, this legal history of surgery since 1740 paraphrases many other documents.)
AHN, Consejos, Leg. 1035, Exp. 1, Parte 5.

Copia de expediente sobre la reforma de la cirugía, enviado al Tribunal del Real Protomedicato, Sept. 7, 1779. (Correspondence between Losada and the Crown, 1776–1779.)
AGS, Gracia y Justicia, Leg. 405.

Copia del expediente del nuevo Colegio de Cirugía de Madrid, división en las tres facultades . . . , y demás incidencias, March 5, 1784. (History of events, including paraphrased documents, between 1768 and 1784.)
AGS, Secretaría de Hacienda, Leg. 549.

*Estatutos . . . que S.M. manda observar a los colegios, y comunidades de cirujanos, establecidos en Barcelona, Cádiz, y en todo el Principado de Cataluña.* Madrid, 1764.
Academia de Medicina, Madrid.

Expediente formado . . . para que las Universidades del Reyno informases por que autores se enseñan todas las Facultades, 1796. (*Informes* of all universities on current curriculum.)
AHM, Consejos, Leg. 5444, Exp. 1.

*Novisima Recopilación de las leyes de España mandada formar por el Señor Don Carlos IV.* 3 vols. Madrid, 1805.

*Ordenanzas de S.M., que deben observarse por el Real Colegio de Cirugía de Barcelona, Cuerpo de Cirugía Militar, colegios subalternos y cirujanos del Principado de Catuluña.* Madrid, 1795.
ARP, Sec. Administriva, Leg. 691.

*Ordenanzas para el gobierno de la cátedra de medicina práctica establecida por S.M. en la Universidad de Valencia.* Madrid, 1797.
AHN, Consejos, Leg. 5444, Exp. 14, Parte 1.

*Ordenanzas que S.M. manda observar por la enseñanza de medicina práctica en las cátedras nuevamente establecidas en el Hospital General de Madrid con la denominación de Estudio Real de Medicina Práctica.* Madrid, 1795.
ARP, Sec. Administriva, Leg. 691.

*Plan de estudios de medicina para la Universidad de Cervera.* Madrid, 1784.
AGS, Gracia y Justicia, Leg. 405.

*Plan de estudios decretado por S.M. en 17 de septiembre de 1845.* Madrid, 1845.

*Plan general de estudios dirigido a la Universidad de Salamanca por el Real y Supremo Consejo de Castilla, y mandado imprimir de su orden.* Salamanca, 1771.
George M. Addy, *The Enlightenment in the University of Salamanca* (Durham, N.C., 1966), pp. 244–366.

*Real Cédula de S.M. y Señores del Consejo, en la cual se fijan las reglas que*

*han de observarse para que se restituya a las universidades y demás establecimientos literarios del Reino la sana enseñanza; y para el abono o inadmisión de los cursos gañados y grados conferidos en ellas en la época del titulado Gobierno Constitucional.* Madrid, 1824.
AHN, Universidades, Sig. 1232.

*Real Cédula de S.M. y Señores del Consejo, en que se aprueban y mandan observar las Ordenanzas formadas para el gobierno económico y escolástico del Colegio de Cirugía establecido en Madrid con el título de San Carlos.* Madrid, 1787.
AHN, Consejos, Leg. 1035, Exp. 1, Parte 1.

*Real Cédula de S.M. y Señores del Consejo, en que se aprueban y mandan observar las Ordenanzas generales formadas para el régimen escolástico y económico de los Reales Colegios de Cirugía, y gobierno de esta Facultad en todo el Reyno.* Madrid, 1804.
AHN, Universidades, Alcalá-Cátedras, Leg. 42, Núm. 74.

*Real Cédula de S.M. y Señores del Consejo, por la cual se manda cesar la Junta General de Gobierno de la Facultad Reunida, se restablece el Protomedicato y que subsista la Junta Superior Gubernativa de Farmacia con lo demás que se expresa.* Madrid, 1801.
AHN, Consejos, Leg. 5444, Exp. 14, Parte 3.

*Real Cédula de S.M. y Señores del Consejo, por la qual se manda formar una Junta Superior de Medicina que vele sobre esta enseñanza, sus progreso y profesores baxo las reglas que se expresan.* Madrid, 1804.
ARP, Sec. Administriva, Leg. 689.

*Real Cédula de S.M. y Señores del Consejo, por la cual se manda observar en todo el Reino el nuevo Reglamento que ha tenido a bien aprobar para el régimen y gobierno de los Colegios de Medicina y Cirugía, y de los profesores que ejerzan estas facultades.* Madrid, 1828.
ARP, Sec. Administriva, Leg. 691.

*Real Cédula de S.M. y Señores del Consejo, por la qual se reduce el número de las universidades literarias del Reyno; se agregan las suprimidas a las que quedan, segun su localidad; y se manda observar en ellas el Plan de Estudios aprobado para la de Salamanca en la forma que se expresa.* Madrid, 1807.
AHN, Universidades, Sig. 1232.

*Reales órdenes expedidas en el año de 1799 por la primera Secretaría de Estado para la reunión del estudio y exercicio de la medicina y cirugía, y erección de una Junta General de Gobierno de esta Facultad Reunida.* Madrid, 1799.
ARP, Sec. Administriva, Leg. 689; AHN, Universidades, Sig. 1232.

Representación de Francisco Antonio de Zunzunegui, 1783. (History of anatomy at the University of Salamanca.)
AHN, Consejos, Leg. 5464, Exp. 14.

## Other Primary Sources

Arrazola, Lorenzo. *Discurso inaugural pronunciado en la solemne apertura de la Universidad Literaria de Madrid.* Madrid, 1845.

*Boletín de medicina, cirugía, y farmacia*, tom. II, 1835.

Bonells, Jaime, and Ignacio Lacaba. *Curso completo de anatomía del cuerpo humano.* 5 vols. Madrid, 1796.

Castelló, Pedro. *Memoria sobre el arreglo de la ciencia de curar que presentó a la Dirección General de Estudios del Reino.* Madrid, 1836.

Castelo Serra, Eusebio. *Biografía del cirujano-médico Pedro Castelló, Marqués de la Salud.* Madrid, 1850.

Corenzo Pérez, José, and Manuel Hermenegildo. *Observaciones sobre el nuevo Plan de Estudios Médicos.* Madrid, 1844.

*Correo de Madrid, o de los Ciegos*, 1787–1790.

Feijóo y Montenegro, Benito Jerónimo. *Cartas eruditas, y curiosas.* 5 vols., 2nd ed. Madrid, 1781.

———. *Teatro crítico.* Edited by Agustín Millares Carlo with an introduction by Gregorio Marañón in *Obras escogidas.* 4 vols. "Biblioteca de Autores Españoles," Vols. 56, 141–143. Madrid, 1863, 1961.

*Gaceta de Madrid*, 1787–1788.

Galli, Leonardi de. *Contestación al informe . . . de las Décadas médico-quirúrgicas y farmacéuticas, o sea justa vindicación de los autores del reglamento del estudio reunido de medicina y cirugía.* Madrid, 1822.

Gimbernat, Agustín de. *Sucinta noticia del S. D. Antonio de Gimbernat.* Barcelona, 1828.

Gimbernat, Antonio de. *Nuevo método de operar en la hernia crural.* Madrid, 1793.

———. *Obras de Don Antonio de Gimbernat precedidas de un estudio biobibliográfico del mismo.* Edited with introduction by Enrique Salcedo y Ginestal. 2 vols. "Biblioteca Clásica de la Medicina Española," Vols. VI–VII. Madrid, 1926–1928.

———. *Oración inaugural que para la abertura de los estudios celebrada en el Real Colegio de Cirugía de Barcelona.* Barcelona, 1768.

Godoy, Manuel. *Memorias críticas y apologéticas.* Edited with introduction by Carlos Seco Serrano. 2 vols. "Biblioteca de Autores Españoles," Vols. 88–89. Madrid, 1956.

González Velasco, Pedro. *Rápida ojeada sobre la anatomía en España.* Madrid, 1856.

*Guía histórica de las universidades, colegios, academias, y demás cuerpos literarios de España y América en que se da noticias de sus fundaciones y estado actual.* Madrid, 1786.

Hernández Morejón, Antonio. *Ensayo de ideología clínica.* Madrid, 1821.

"Informe del Claustro de Medicina de Valencia sobre renovación de estudios

[1721]," *Archivo Iberoamericano de Historia de la Medicina y Antropología Médica*, XIII (1961), 143–155.

*Instrucciones generales sobre el orden y método de enseñanza en las Facultades Médicas del Reino*. Madrid, 1846.

Jovellanos, Gaspar Melchor de. *Obras de D. Gaspar Melchor de Jovellanos.* Edited with introduction by Candido Nocedal and Miguel Artola. 5 vols. "Biblioteca de Autores Españoles," Vols. 46, 50, 85–87. Madrid, 1858, 1956.

La Forest, Comte de. *Correspondance du Comte de la Forest.* Edited by Geoffroy de Grandmaison. 7 vols. Paris, 1908.

*Memorial literario instructivo y curioso de la Corte de Madrid*, 1784–1790.

*Memorias de la Real Academia Médica de Madrid*, tom. I, 1797.

Olavide, Pablo de. *Plan de estudios para la Universidad de Sevilla.* With an introduction by Francisco Aguilar Pinal. Barcelona, 1969.

Pérez de Escobar, Antonio. *Medicina patria o elementos de la medicina práctica de Madrid.* Madrid, 1788.

Sánchez de Toca, Melchor. *Memoria sobre el Plan de Estudios, la organización y el personal de las escuelas médicas estranjeras con aplicaciones a la nacional de San Carlos de Madrid.* Madrid, 1840.

Seoane, Mateo. *El nuevo plan de estudios médicos.* Madrid, 1843.

Velasco Ceballos, Romulo (ed.). *La cirugía mexicana en el siglo XVIII.* Mexico City, 1946.

## Secondary Sources

Ackerknecht, Erwin H. *Medicine at the Paris Hospital, 1794–1848.* Baltimore, 1967.

———. *A Short History of Medicine.* New York, 1955.

Addy, George M. *The Enlightenment in the University of Salamanca.* Durham, N.C., 1966.

Aguilar Piñal, Francisco. *La Universidad de Sevilla en el siglo XVIII: Estudio sobre la primera reforma universitaria moderna.* Seville, 1969.

Ajo González y Sáinz de Zúñiga, C. M. *Historia de las universidades hispánicas: orígines y desarrollo desde su aparición a nuestros días.* 5 vols. Madrid, 1957–1966.

Alcázar Molina, Cayetano. "El despotismo ilustrado en España," *Bulletin of the International Committee of Historical Sciences*, V (1933), 727–751.

Aldridge, A. Owen (ed.). *The Ibero-American Enlightenment.* Urbana, Ill., 1971.

Alonso Muñoyerro, Luis. *La Facultad de Medicina en la Universidad de Alcalá de Henares.* Madrid, 1945.

Alvarez de Morales, Antonio. *La "Ilustración" y la reforma de la Universidad en la España del siglo XVIII.* Madrid, 1971.

Alvarez Requejo, Felipe. *El Conde de Campomanes: Su obra histórica.* Oviedo, 1954.

Alvarez-Sierra, José. *Carlos III y la higiene pública.* Madrid, 1956.

———. *Historia de la cirugía española.* Madrid, 1961.

Aparicio Simón, José. *Historia del Real Colegio de San Carlos de Madrid.* Madrid, 1956.

Artola Gallego, Miguel. *Los afrancesados.* Madrid, 1958.

———. *La España de Fernando VII.* With introduction by Carlos Seco Serrano. (Ramón Menéndez Pidal, "Historia de España," Vol. XXVI.) Madrid, 1968.

———. *Los orígenes de la España contemporánea.* 2 vols. Madrid, 1959.

Atkinson, William C. *A History of Spain and Portugal.* Baltimore, 1960.

Ballesteros y Beretta. *Historia de España y su influencia en la historia universal,* 10 vols., 2nd ed., rev. Madrid, 1958.

Barriola, Ignacio María. *Los Amigos del País y la medicina.* San Sebastián, 1963.

Beltrán de Heredia, R. P. *Los orígenes de la Universidad de Salamanca.* Salamanca, 1953.

British Congress on the History of Medicine. *The Evolution of Medical Education in Britain.* Edited by F. N. L. Poynter. London, 1966.

Butterfield, Herbert. *The Origins of Modern Science.* 2nd ed., rev. New York, 1957.

Callahan, William J. *Honor, Commerce, and Industry in Eighteenth-Century Spain.* Boston, 1972.

Callega, Julián. *Breves noticias de la Facultad de Medicina de Madrid.* Madrid, 1876.

Carr, Raymond. *Spain, 1808–1939.* Oxford, 1966.

Carreras y Artau, Tomás. *Estudios sobre médicos-filósofos españoles del siglo XIX.* Barcelona, 1952.

Cartwright, Frederick F. *The Development of Modern Surgery.* New York, 1967.

Cassirer, Ernst. *The Philosophy of the Enlightenment.* Translated by Fritz C. A. Koelln and James P. Pettegrove. Princeton, 1951.

Castiglioni, Arturo. *A History of Medicine.* Translated and edited by E. B. Krumbhaar. New York, 1941.

Chastenet, Jacques. *Godoy, Master of Spain, 1792–1808.* Translated by J. F. Huntington. London, 1953.

Cope, Zachary. *The Royal College of Surgeons of England.* Springfield, Ill., 1959.

Corona, Carlos. *Revolución y reacción en el reinado de Carlos IV.* Madrid, 1957.

Creswell, Clarendon Hyde. *The Royal College of Surgeons of Edinburgh, 1505–1905.* Edinburgh, 1926.

Defourneaux, Marcelin. *Pablo de Olavide, el afrancesado.* Translated by Manuel Martínez Camaró. Mexico City, 1965.

Desdevises du Dezert, Georges. "Les Institutions de l'Espagne au XVIIIe Siècle," *Revue Hispanique*, LXX (1927), 1–556.

———. "La Richesse et la Civilisation Espagnole au XVIIIe Siècle," *Revue Hispanique*, LXXIII (1928), 1–488.

———. "La Société Espagnole au XVIIIe Siècle," *Revue Hispanique*, LXIV (1925), 225–654.

Díaz-Plaja, Fernando. *La vida española en el siglo XVIII.* Barcelona, 1946.

———. *La vida española en el siglo XIX.* Madrid, 1952.

Domínguez Ortiz, Antonio. *La sociedad española en el siglo XVIII.* Madrid, 1955.

*Dorland's Illustrated Medical Dictionary.* 23rd ed. Philadelphia, 1957.

Dulieu, Louis. "Pierre Chirac, sa vie, ses écrits, ses idées," *Montpellier Medical*, 3rd ser., LI (1957), 767–786.

Espinosa y González-Pérez, Francisco. "El Conde de Aranda," *La España moderna*, XXI (1909), 5–18.

Fehrenbach, Charles Wentz. "Moderados and Exaltados: The Liberal Opposition to Ferdinand VII, 1814–1823," *Hispanic American Historical Review*, L (1970), 52–69.

Fernández del Castillo, Francisco. *La Facultad de Medicina según el Archivo de la Real y Pontificia Universidad de México.* Mexico City, 1953.

Ferrer, Diego. *Historia del Real Colegio de Cirugía de la Armada de Cádiz.* Cádiz, 1961.

Ferrer del Rio, Antonio. *Historia del reinado de Carlos III en España.* 4 vols. Madrid, 1856.

Fontana Lazaro, Josep. *La quiebra de la monarquía absoluta, 1814–1820.* Barcelona, 1971.

García del Real, Eduardo. *Historia de la medicina en España.* Madrid, 1921.

Garrison, Fielding H. *An Introduction to the History of Medicine.* 4th ed., rev. Philadelphia, 1929.

Gay, Peter. *The Enlightenment: An Interpretation.* 2 vols. New York, 1966, 1969.

Gelfand, Toby. "Empiricism and Eighteenth-Century French Surgery," *Bulletin of the History of Medicine, XLIV* (1973), 40–53.

———. "From Guild to Profession: The Surgeons of France in the 18th Century," *Texas Reports on Biology and Medicine*, XXXII (1974), 121–134.

———. "The Hospice of the Paris College of Surgery (1774–1793), 'A Unique and Valuable Institution,' " *Bulletin of the History of Medicine*, XLVII (1973), 375–393.

———. "The 'Paris Manner' of Dissection: Student Anatomical Dissection in Early Eighteenth-Century Paris," *Bulletin of the History of Medicine*, XLVI (1972), 99–130.

———. "The Training of Surgeons in Eighteenth-Century Paris and Its Influence on Medical Education." Unpublished Ph.D. dissertation, The Johns Hopkins University, 1973.

Gutiérrez Galdo, José. "Los planes de estudios de la Facultad de Medicina de Granada en los siglos XVI, XVII, y XVIII," *Actualidad Médica*, XLI (Aug. 1965), 643–655.

Hahn, Roger. *The Anatomy of Scientific Institutions: The Paris Academy of Sciences, 1666–1803*. Berkeley, 1971.

Hall, Courtney R. "The Rise of Professional Surgery in the United States, 1800–1865," *Bulletin of the History of Medicine*, XXVI (1952), 231–262.

Hamilton, Earl J. *War and Prices in Spain, 1651–1800*. Cambridge, Mass., 1947.

Hartzenbusch, Eugenio. *Apuntes para un catálogo de periódicos madrileños desde 1661 al 1870*. Madrid, 1894.

Haviland, Thomas N., and Lawrence C. Parish. "A Brief Account of the Use of Wax Models in the Study of Medicine," *Journal of the History of Medicine and Allied Sciences*, XXV (1970), 52–75.

Hazard, Paul. *European Thought in the Eighteenth Century from Montesquieu to Lessing*. Translated by J. Lewis May. Cleveland, 1963.

Hernández Morejón, Antonio. *Historia bibliográfica de la medicina española*. 7 vols. Madrid, 1842–1852.

Herr, Richard. *The Eighteenth Century Revolution in Spain*. Princeton, 1958.

Horn, D. B. *A Short History of the University of Edinburgh, 1556–1889*. Edinburgh, 1967.

Iborra, Pascual. "Memoria sobre la institución del Real Proto-Medicato," *Anales de la Real Academia de Medicina*, VI (1885–1886), 183–307, 387–397, 531–532, 570–592.

Kagan, Richard L. *Students and Society in Early Modern Spain*. Baltimore, 1974.

———. "Universities in Castile, 1500–1700," *Past and Present*, No. 49 (Nov. 1970), pp. 44–71.

———. "Universities in Castile, 1500–1810," in Lawrence Stone (ed.), *University in Society*, Vol. II. Princeton, 1974.

Kamen, Henry. *The Spanish Inquisition*. New York, 1965.

Kany, Charles E. *Life and Manners in Madrid, 1750–1800*. Berkeley, 1932.

King, Lester S. *The Growth of Medical Thought*. Chicago, 1963.

———. "Medical Theory and Practice at the Beginning of the 18th Century," *Bulletin of the History of Medicine*, XLVI (1972), 1–15.

———. *The Medical World of the Eighteenth Century*. Chicago, 1958.

Krebs Wilckens, Ricardo. *El pensamiento histórico, político, y económico del Conde de Campomanes*. Santiago, Chile, 1960.

La Fuente, Vicente de. *Historia de las universidades, colegios, y demás establecimientos de enseñanza en España*. 4 vols. Madrid, 1884–1889.

Laín Entralgo, Pedro. *Historia de la medicina moderna y contemporánea.* 2nd ed. Barcelona, 1963.

Lanning, John Tate. *The Eighteenth-Century Enlightenment in the University of San Carlos de Guatemala.* Ithaca, N.Y., 1956.

———. "Legitimacy and *Limpieza de Sangre* in the Practice of Medicine in the Spanish Empire," *Jahrbuch für Geschichte von Staat, Wirtschaft und Gesellschaft Lateinamerikas*, IV (1967), 37–60.

———. "Tradition and the Enlightenment in the Spanish Colonial Universities," *Cahiers d'Histoire Mondiale*, X (1967), 705–721.

———. *The University in the Kingdom of Guatemala.* Ithaca, N.Y., 1955.

Lapuente Mateos, Alfredo. "La fundación del Real Colegio de Cirugía de San Carlos," *Revista mensual de ciencias médicas*, XIV (1946), 1–22.

———. "Juntas literarias y censuras en el Real Colegio de San Carlos," *Archivos iberoamericanos de historia de la medicina*, I (1949), 408–418.

———. "Para la historia de la Hermandad de San Cosme y San Damian," *Medicamenta*, IX (Jan. 1948), 97.

Leonardo, Richard A. *History of Surgery.* New York, 1943.

Lindeboom, G. A. *Herman Boerhaave: The Man and His Work.* London, 1968.

López Piñero, José María. "Harvey's Doctrine of the Blood in Seventeenth-Century Spain," *Journal of the History of Medicine and Allied Sciences*, XXVIII (1973), 230–242.

Lovett, Gabriel H. *Napoleon and the Birth of Modern Spain.* 2 vols. New York, 1965.

Madol, Hans Roger. *Godoy, el primer dictador de nuestro tiempo.* Translated by A. Sans Huelin and M. Sandmann. Madrid, 1966.

Malo y Calvo, Joaquín. *Reseña histórica de la biblioteca de la Facultad de Medicina de Madrid.* Madrid, 1875.

Martínez Durán, Carlos. *Las ciencias médicas en Guatemala.* 3rd ed. Guatemala City, 1964.

Menéndez y Pelayo, Marcelino. *La ciencia española.* Edited by Enrique Sánchez Reyes. 3 vols. ("Obras completas," vols. 58–91). Madrid, 1953–1954.

Mercader Riba, Juan, and Antonio Domínguez Ortiz. "La época del despotismo ilustrado," in Jaime Vicens Vives (ed.), *Historia social y económica de España y América*, Vol. IV. 2nd edition. Madrid, 1971.

Moll, Aristides A. *Aesculapius in Latin America.* Philadelphia, 1944.

Motten, Clement G. *Mexican Silver and the Enlightenment.* Philadelphia, 1950.

Muñoyerro, Luis Alonso. *La Facultad de Medicina en la Universidad de Alcalá de Henares.* Madrid, 1945.

Muñoz Pérez, José. "La España de Carlos III y su conciencia de período histórico," *Estudios sobre historia de España.* Edited by Manuel Fernández Alvarez. Madrid, 1965.

Nasio, Juan. "La ciencia médica hispánica en los siglos XVI, XVII, y XVIII y su contraste con la ciencia extranjera," *Medicamenta,* XXIII (1955), 221–224.

Norwood, William F. "Medicine in the Era of the American Revolution," *International Record of Medicine,* LXXI (1958), 391–407.

O'Malley, C. D. (ed.). *The History of Medical Education.* "UCLA Forum in Medical Sciences," No. 12. Los Angeles, 1970.

Payne, Stanley G. *A History of Spain and Portugal.* 2 vols. Madison, Wis., 1973.

Peset Reig, Mariano, and José Luis Peset Reig. *El reformismo de Carlos III y la Universidad de Salamanca.* Salamanca, 1969.

———. *La universidad española (siglos XVIII y XIX): Despotismo ilustrado y revolución liberal.* Madrid, 1974.

Polt, John H. R. *Jovellanos and His English Sources.* Philadelphia, 1965.

Postell, William D. "Medical Education and Medical Schools in Colonial America," *International Record of Medicine,* LXXI (1958), 364–376.

Puschmann, Theodor. *A History of Medical Education.* Translated and edited by Evan H. Hare. London, 1891.

Reglá Campistol, Juan, and Santiago Alcolea. *El Siglo XVIII.* Barcelona, 1957.

Rodríguez Casado, Vicente. "Iglesia y estado en el reinado de Carlos III," *Estudios americanos,* I (1948), 5–57.

———. *La política y los políticos en el reinado de Carlos III.* Madrid, 1962.

Rudé, George. *Europe in the Eighteenth Century.* New York, 1973.

Sánchez Agesta, Luis. *El pensamiento político del despotismo ilustrado.* Madrid, 1953.

Sánchez Granjel, Luis. *Anatomía española de la ilustración.* "Cuadernos de Historia de la Medicina Española," Vol. I. Salamanca, 1963.

———. *Historia de la medicina española.* Barcelona, 1962.

Sanvisens Marfull, Alejandro. *Un médico-filósofo español del siglo XVIII: El Doctor Andrés Piquer.* Barcelona, 1953.

Sarrablo Aguareles, Eugenio. *La vida en Madrid durante la ocupación francesa de 1808 a 1813.* Zaragoza, 1964.

Sarrailh, Jean. *La España ilustrada de la segunda mitad del siglo XVIII.* Translated by Antonio Alatorre. Mexico City, 1957.

Schulte, Henry F. *The Spanish Press, 1470–1966: Print, Power, and Politics.* Urbana, Ill., 1968.

Serrano Poncela, Segundo. "Godoy y los ilustrados," *Formas de vida hispánica.* Madrid, 1963.

Shafer, Robert Jones. *The Economic Societies in the Spanish World.* Syracuse, N.Y., 1958.

Shryock, Richard Harrison. *The Development of Modern Medicine*. Philadelphia, 1936.

Sigerist, Henry E. *Civilization and Disease*. Phoenix Science Series. Chicago, 1943.

———. *A History of Medicine*. 2 vols. New York, 1951, 1961.

———. *Henry E. Sigerist on the History of Medicine*. Edited with introduction by Felix Martí-Ibánez. New York, 1960.

Singer, Charles, and E. Ashworth Underwood. *A Short History of Medicine*. New York, 1962.

Snapper, I. *Meditations on Medicine and Medical Education*. New York, 1956.

Soroa y Pineda, Antonio. "El Hospital General de Madrid como escuela, templo, tradición y fortaleza señera de la medicina de la villa y corte," *Gaceta médica española*, XXXVIII (1964), 337–342.

Suárez, Federico. "Fernando VII," *Estudios americanos*, IV (1952), 5–25.

Tapia Ozcariz, Enrique de. *Carlos III y su época*. Madrid, 1962.

Temkin, Owsei. *Galenism: Rise and Decline of a Medical Philosophy*. Ithaca, N.Y., 1973.

———. "The Role of Surgery in the Rise of Modern Medical Thought," *Bulletin of the History of Medicine*, XXV (1951), 248–259.

Trevor-Roper, H. R. "The Spanish Enlightenment," *The Times Literary Supplement*, March 15, 1957, pp. 153–155.

Tuñon de Lara, Manuel. *La España del Siglo XIX*. Paris, 1961.

Turner, A. Logan. *Story of a Great Hospital: The Royal Infirmary of Edinburgh, 1726–1929*. Edinburgh, 1937.

Usandizaga, Manuel. *Historia del Real Colegio de Cirugía de San Carlos de Madrid*. Madrid, 1948.

Villa, Julián de la. "Historia del Hospital General, hoy Provincial," *Anales de la Real Academia Nacional de Medicina*, LXXIII (1956), 51–61.

Voltes, Pedro. *Carlos III y su tiempo*. Barcelona, 1964.

Wall, Cecil. *The History of the Surgeon's Company, 1745–1800*. London, 1937.

Whitaker, Arthur P. "Changing and Unchanging Interpretations of the Enlightenment in Spanish America," *Proceedings of the American Philosophical Society*, CXIV (Aug. 1970), 256–271.

———. "The Elhuyar Mining Mission and the Enlightenment," *Hispanic American Historical Review*, XXXI (1951), 556–585.

Williams, L. P. "Science, Education, and Napoleon," *Isis*, XLVII (1956), 369–382.

Wolf, A. *A History of Science, Technology, and Philosophy in the Eighteenth Century*. New York, 1939.

Zaragoza Rubira, Juan Ramón. "Los hospitales españoles en el primer tercio del siglo XIX," *Medicina española*, XLVIII (1962), 149–158.

# Index